(longer during
COVID-19
lockdown)

Diary of a Modern

Consumptive

PAUL THORN

TO WHOM IT SHOULD CONCERN

This book is dedicated to the millions of individuals who have died of tuberculosis (TB) throughout the centuries. To those with the disease who are sick today, stay strong. To those who will needlessly perish in the future if we don't provide the resources, healthcare systems, new and affordable high-quality life-saving drugs, not only to manage and cure TB, but also humanely to eradicate it for good, I simply ask the question, "Why"? I directly appeal to the leaders of the world to achieve what is possible – in our lifetime, a world finally free from TB.

CONTENTS

Acknowledgments   7

1   Foreword by Jennifer Furin, MD., PhD.   9

2   Jack O'Sullivan, *The Independent*, 1999   15

3   Introduction   17

4   Nocturne – Prologue   23

5   Part 1: Infection   31

    Part 2: Cure   49

6   Diurne – Epilogue   145

ACKNOWLEDGMENTS

There are many to whom I owe my sincere gratitude and thanks. Firstly, to Mark King, who designed the book cover, and Bryony Weaver for her editing skills. To the few who stood by me when I, and everyone else, believed I was dying, who sat with me in that darkest of times and held my hand. To the doctors and nurses at St. Mary's Hospital who cared for me and never gave up, even when I was at my most trying. Extra-special thanks to those who took the time to write letters to me, even though they didn't know me personally, but who became aware of my situation. Thank you for giving me strength and hope – and for restoring some of my faith in humanity.

FOREWORD

JENNIFER FURIN, MD., PhD.

Harvard Medical School, Department of

Global Health and Social Medicine

Isolation. It is a word with multiple meanings. In medical parlance it is a term used to describe the process by which someone with a transmissible infectious disease is removed from the larger community and placed in a setting where he or she receives treatment until there is no longer a risk of the disease being spread to the general public. Often viewed as a necessary and important public health protection, entire hospital wards and facilities are built for the purposes of medical isolation. But the term isolation also has a social meaning. It is used to describe the profound loneliness an individual experiences when he or she is removed from social networks and participation in the richness of human interactions. It can leave a person deserted, depressed, and wondering whether life is worth living.

These medical and social concepts of isolation are often at war with one another, pitting a "greater good" against an individual's misery. Nowhere is this better illustrated than with the disease of tuberculosis (TB). Human beings have long wrestled with *Mycobacterium tuberculosis*, the pathogen that causes TB. First identified in Peruvian mummies, TB today is the leading cause of death from an infectious disease in adults. An estimated 10.4 million new people fall sick with TB each year, of whom at least 1.7 million die of the disease. Drug-resistant forms of TB—which require treatment with prolonged and toxic regimens that are only able to cure about 50% of those who receive them—are also on the rise and are poised to be the leading cause of death due to antimicrobial resistance. TB, in whatever form it comes, is a horror that nobody should have to face: it is characterized by fever, coughing (oftentimes blood), and a weight loss so profound that it has been given the colloquial name of "consumption", since the body is often left skeletal and wasted by the disease. It is also characterized by stigma, discrimination, and an imposed solitude that is said to consume the soul.

The experience of this devastating illness is the subject of Paul Thorn's riveting biography, *Diary of a Modern Consumptive*. In the living pages of this book, we are given a first-hand account of what it is like to live in isolation while battling with a mortal disease. It is a shattering story of the failures of modern medicine when it comes to TB. It is also, however, a miraculous memoir documenting the power of human connectedness even in the face of severe and imposed confinement.

Although the book is about isolation, Paul's journey is not an isolated event. Even now, millions of individuals face the same catastrophic experiences he eloquently describes. Much of shared suffering can be attributed to the way the global community has responded to the problem of TB using a public health approach. The public health approach— usually sold as a means of achieving the best results for the most people at the lowest cost—is a weapon often wielded in the war against infectious diseases. While there may be some merits to conceptualizing and responding to the world's plagues in such a fashion, the public health approach is also incredibly dehumanizing. It sacrifices the pain of individual people on the altar of benefit to an often-abstract human mass. And to date, this public health approach to TB has failed, as seen in the dismal global statistics, the lack of new diagnostic and treatment tools, and the planned exclusion of vulnerable populations, most notably children.

There is, however, an alternative TB strategy that could finally turn the tide against this age-old scourge: a human-rights based approach to the disease. Paul provides a blueprint for such an approach in his diary, which stresses the significance of each person's unique journey with TB. A human rights-based approach to TB means putting the person with TB at the center of all activities and striving to achieve the best possible outcome for every single man, woman, and child who is affected by the disease. It means that all people with TB - regardless of their geographic location or perceived level in society - should be offered the most sensitive diagnostic tests, be treated with the most effective medicines, be provided with all the means to prevent the development of TB, and receive care in a way that allows them to continue to live dignified and productive lives. It does not view the provision of such services as extravagant extras but rather as fundamental basics that form the core of the management of TB. Most importantly, the human-rights based approach to TB is characterized by a lack of external discrimination and internal shame—hallmarks of TB to this very day—as people living with the disease are transformed into the respected and insightful leaders they are, possessing the collective wisdom needed to once and for all stop this deadly disease. Isolated no more, they will be the driving force that may finally allow us to put TB in the past where it belongs.

Jennifer Furin, MD., PhD. (2018)

"When you meet Paul for the first time, you wonder whether you are really in his home or in a hospital ward. I have just stepped off the street from the blaze of color that is London's Chinatown. Yet this haven is devoted to an antiseptic life. The walls are a clinical white. There are no curtains, no carpets, just well-polished wooden floors. The central light, modelled on a Sputnik spacecraft, would look well in an operating theatre. There are no books, just piles of file boxes that could contain patient's notes.

And then there is the individual himself, swallowed up in this whiteness. Paul looks drawn and tired. You can almost hear Keats's own angry line against the ravages of tuberculosis: "Youth grows pale and spectre thin and dies."

He caught a particularly nasty strain of TB, resistant to all but the most toxic drugs... seven others are dead. How did Paul survive? - It led him to write, detailing a descent into despair after one doctor warned him that he might never leave the isolation room alive..."

Jack O'Sullivan, *The Independent*, 1999

INTRODUCTION

I've been HIV-positive since 1988, and I was 17 years old when I was infected. In 1995, as I was becoming ill with an AIDS-related illness, I was infected with Multidrug-resistant tuberculosis (MDR-TB). If you read between the lines of this book you will see that I'm more than a virus or disease. I'm a human being, full of hopes and dreams and prone to fear like everyone else. As I write now, it is 2018. There's still, hopefully, a lot of life to live.

I was a patient on an HIV unit at a West London hospital when I contracted MDR-TB. The outbreak occurred when staff didn't follow infection-control procedures. They carried out several induced sputum sample tests on a patient who had come from Brazil (via Portugal) on the open ward where we were also situated. Inducing sputum is a simple procedure whereby the patient breathes in vaporized salty water (saline) so that he coughs, and sputum samples can be collected for testing. We should never have been in the same room as him whilst the procedure was carried out. Consequently, seven others, including me, breathed in the infectious bacterium that he coughed up. I am the sole survivor of this oversight of safe procedure.

For some time prior to my experience, experts had been predicting that it was only a matter of time before an outbreak of TB/MDR-TB occurred in such a way on an HIV unit.

Three months after exposure to the potentially deadly bacteria, I was told of the "accident" on the HIV unit. My health had already been deteriorating prior to my knowledge of the event. During that time, the bacilli multiplied slowly in my lungs without me knowing. My slowly-advancing chest pain and breathlessness was finally explained. Then, without warning, I lost my liberty and was locked away from society in a negative-pressure isolation room so that I didn't infect anyone else. I was told it was probable I would never leave, and to prepare to die. I was aged 24 and my short life was seemingly over.

I kept a diary detailing my decline to the ravages of this age-old adversary. This work, *Diary of a*

Modern Consumptive, is an edited collection of my diary entries, quotes from media coverage that occurred in response to the outbreak at the time and correspondence that was sent to me, often by people I'd never have the pleasure to meet or know. They are brought together here to tell my story. It's by no means unique, and it could have been told millions of times before by those who have already exhaled their last. Voices lost to the march of time. The book documents how I was infected, the diagnosis, the loneliness of isolation, about the masked and faceless people who were caring for me, the hardships of having to take toxic drugs and their side effects, and my eventual cure.

The inspiration behind this book is the work of 'consumptive' writers now long gone: John Keats, the Brontë sisters, D.H. Lawrence, Robert Louis Stevenson, George Orwell, Katherine Mansfield and countless others. There are hundreds of probably more excellent quotations by 'consumptive' writers in literary history that I could have used in this book. Personally, I identify very much with Katherine Mansfield and have taken the liberty of using those of her quotations that resonate with me.

Mansfield was born in New Zealand on October

14th, 1888. She was a prominent short-story writer, although she is also known for her diaries and letters. At 19, she settled in the United Kingdom, where she became a friend of writers such as D.H. Lawrence and Virginia Woolf. In 1917, she was diagnosed with TB, which eventually led to her death in Fontainebleau-Avon, France, in 1923.

Although I have no right whatsoever to compare myself with Mansfield as a writer, I do relate to her unconventional lifestyle, which, even by today's standards nearly a century later, might raise an eyebrow or two! I identify with her hopes and fears, her vulnerability and strength. I have a level of understanding of the quotations I've used in this short book, which many who have survived TB will also recognize in themselves. For Mansfield and many other writers and artists, having TB inspired their work, and indeed, it defined a whole era when many great writers and artists seemed to have TB. There were even those who thought that to be truly creative, a writer must be 'consumptive' – pale and febrile, coughing blood into a lace handkerchief, suffering for their art to create any work of merit. It's a romantic notion, but the reality can't be more different.

So, why has it taken me so long to write this book, more than two decades since the events of 1995? Like myself, my journals and letters pertaining to the time I had MDR-TB nearly didn't survive. In November 2006, I stood over a bonfire, throwing years of work into the flames. To me it was a symbolic gesture as I looked forward to a new future made possible by the miracle of managing HIV with anti-retroviral drugs. The ashes of my journals, a couple of hundred notebooks in total, were still smoldering two days after I had set light to them.

However, not all my journals met this fate. When it came to sending the volumes relating to 1995, detailing my experience of having MDR-TB into the flames, I hesitated. I've wanted to write this book for some time, but the problem had been that I couldn't face reading them again in any detail. I kept making excuses and stalling. I'd really tried to give up on the idea of writing this book, but the idea had only gotten stronger over time. I wondered, if I finally destroyed the journals, would the unwritten book that had been nagging me for more than two decades ever leave me alone? Being haunted by it indefinitely was not a chance I wanted to take.

I've thought long and hard about how to write

this book. Indeed, I experimented with several ways of presenting it, laying down words only to decide that I wasn't happy with the finished book. I hope I've created something that works! Also, my surname used to be Mayho. I changed it by deed poll in 2003. The newspaper reports also quoted in this book refer to me by my name at the time. I am, however, still the same person.

There were times when writing this book was very difficult, especially when reading again my journals and the letters that were sent me. I thought about relighting the bonfire and consigning the whole lot to the flames. But if you have TB or MDR-TB and this book brings you hope, then I'm very glad I didn't.

Paul Thorn (2018)

NOCTURNE - PROLOGUE

"I sometimes wonder whether the act of surrender is not one of the greatest of them all – the highest. It is one of the (most) difficult of all... it is so immensely complicated. It 'needs' real humility and at the same time an absolute belief in one's own essential freedom. It is an act of faith. At the last moments like all great acts it is pure risk."

The Letters of Katherine Mansfield

My world has become very small; a room with a bed, a chair and a window with metal bars. The stench of the dirty drain from the shower is filling my nostrils. There's no solace from it and nowhere to escape to. I turn my mind outwards, trying to imagine the world beyond the anti-chamber's two closed doors that separate me from a different, more pleasant reality. Lying back and looking at the ceiling, I wonder if it will be the last thing that I will ever see? Younger than John Keats, who knew he was dying on seeing the red arterial blood in his handkerchief, youth truly is spectre-thin and pale, and by all accounts I am going to die. The doctor had told me, so it must be true. There's little, it seems, I can do. Powerless. I close my eyes and my mind wanders somewhere between consciousness and sleep.

I now understand, like millions before me, why they used to call tuberculosis 'consumption'. Ravaged by fever and drenched in sweat, I can feel my life ebbing away and being gently soaked up by the sheets that I lie in. Unlike the solitude one chooses, my isolation has been forced upon me. There is no choice in the matter. It is for your protection that I must remain separate from you.

The days no longer have a beginning or an end, melding together. I wake to find myself in the same place again. Feeling like it's someone else's life and not my own. A surge of the fear of dying, the only punctuation in what essentially is the same moment in time over and over. I do nothing, except write, and I go nowhere, except for the sanctuary of my diary.

I can see the fear in their eyes as they try to breathe with waspish breaths inside the orange facemasks meant to protect them from me. Only in my dreams do I escape them, these people with faces I never see. But the waking hours seem crueler than they are. The clock on the wall laboriously ticks without me counting the seconds that go by, but I can feel the space in between each one as the tuberculosis bacilli take advantage of those mounting gaps, replicating slowly inside me.

Does true surrender come when one admits that death is as natural as being born? What do you want of me says the host? With me surely you shall die too? One thing is certain in all of this and is clear to me now. We humans are united in the air that we breathe, whatever our differences, and ultimately in death, whenever that comes. The great equalizer.

How does a young man, only 24 years old, accept the inevitability of his death, hostage to a disease that has already stalked the world for thousands of years, and that has taken some of humanity's finest? Stripping away everything until the host, finally ethereally pale, a shadow of how they used to be, becomes translucent in physicality and spirit, before finally and begrudgingly letting go of his soul. I am not ready for that most final of acts, that of surrender. I just can't. I don't want to die.

Five years before, on September 3rd, 1990, I was diagnosed HIV-positive. It was not a good day to be diagnosed. Not that any given day is. It was the day that Florida dentist David Acer died. He infamously had infected five of his patients, including a 16-year-old girl with the virus. They were either already dead or dying. The public were frightened. Could it really be possible that those we entrusted with our lives, who were supposed to care for us, might potentially transmit a disease that could kill us? I was a student nurse back then, young, starting out in life and learning the skills for a future that feels now to have been snatched away from me. Needless to say, being diagnosed HIV-positive was the end of my nursing career. I would care for no one (professionally) again, and it was my turn to take the place of the patient and be cared for by the 'professionals'. Like the 'public', whatever that word means in its loosest term, I didn't think that the actions of those to whom I'd entrusted my care would have led me to being infected with a disease that could kill me, led me to the predicament I find myself in now within these walls, isolated in this room.

The bacterial bouquet grown in a Petri dish may well have excited the observer in his or her white coat, as he/ she looked at it though his microscope, but does that excitement, their interest in me as a disease, not as a person, mean anything to anyone but them?

Only a few years after being diagnosed HIV-positive I was becoming ill, and my admissions to hospital were becoming more frequent. It was during one of these stays that I became infected with MDR-TB. The prognosis for me is not good; I was told that most HIV-positive people who have MDR-TB usually die. My doctor thinks I may have only three months to live.

I, like you, probably, thought that TB had been eradicated. Not so. Humanity's triumph over the microbe and the miracle of antibiotics was short-lived, it seems. TB, in my mind, belonged to a time more than a century ago when famous writers experimented with opiates and drank Absinthe into dream-addled oblivion.

It's a fact that I am sure you won't dispute; literature is scattered with the great works of 'consumptive' writers. There was a time when if a writer wasn't consumptive, then he or she really couldn't be taken seriously. They just weren't pale and interesting enough. At least I have that credential, if nothing else.

Keeping in mind that the written works of those who were inspired to write *because* they were 'consumptive' tend to hang around for some time – like I say, you may have heard of Keats, the Brontës, Mansfield etc., right? I shan't labour the point – I feel it important to explain something to you. After all, I could be dead as you read this, and I'd hate to seem so self-referential as to compare myself to those great writers. They lived in seemingly more romantic times, enhanced strangely by TB, and pioneers, if you will, of the 'consumptive' art form.

No, the link between those writers and me is keeping a diary. For me, it's the 'place' where I go to externalise the contents of my mind and imagination, allowing it to wander freely, and now it seems to make sense of the tragedy of a life cut short.

Those masked jailers caring for me have shut the door and are waiting for me to drown on the bloody contents of my lungs. Is it too late? The realisation is that I've already wasted enough time waiting to die – it's been several years since my HIV diagnosis. Now I realise that I should have 'lived' those years, not in fear but in liberty and freedom, not experiencing repeatedly the pain of my past, but enjoying the world around me, my friends, my lovers and those who truly care about me. What now? What can I do in such a short future? There's no time left for regrets.

I wake from the dampness of my night sweat. At least, I think I have... I'm a bit more lucid now. I had a dream. I dreamt that everything I'd ever written, everything I'd ever said, thought or done was documented on a long tape of thin, white paper. The thin paper ribbon hung out of my mouth and I started to pull it out. Out with it came piles of the tape which started to form on the floor as I continued to tug away at it. I did this for a long time, and then the tape snapped. There was still some poking from my lips and I pulled it again, but this time it wouldn't move. I slid it from side to side in the hope that it would be released and continue to flow, but it would not. I knew there was a lot more down inside me and I wanted it out, but I feared that if I pulled too hard and the tape snapped further down my throat, I wouldn't be able to draw it out at all. I sat there, not knowing what to do. Everything I knew, consciously or subconsciously, was in there. I had to have courage – I would just have to risk breaking it.

PART 1 - INFECTION

"...All I am doing now is trying to put into practice the 'ideas' I have had for so long, of another and far more truthful existence. I want to learn something that no books can teach me, and I want to try and escape from my terrible illness. That again you can't be expected to understand. You think I am like other people – I mean, normal. I'm not. I don't know which is the ill me and which is the well me. I am simply one pretence after another. Only now I recognise it..."

The Letters of Katherine Mansfield (Written less than three months before her death from TB in Fontainebleau-Avon, France, January 9th, 1923.)

[Diary] Saturday 8th April, 1995

I just have to accept that being ill is part and parcel of

being HIV-positive. I find myself in hospital again with another infection. It's not anything that they can put a name to, just one of those stomach bugs that are real stubborn and hard to get rid of.

I've been on this ward a few times. This time around, I'm on a bay in which there are six beds. I'm in the bed closest to the main entrance of the ward. I can see the nurses at their station from here. Opposite me is a man who is clearly very ill. He's very thin, and it's a look I've seen before. It's nearly his time. He coughs throughout the day and night. It keeps me awake. I know he can't help it, but I'm tired and my thoughts aren't kind. I feel ashamed that I mutter to myself that he should just get on with it and die so the rest of us can get some sleep. It's selfish I know, and when I'm more awake I'm capable of the compassion this young man deserves.

I had some visitors today. Their white habits and crucifixes were a sight to see as they walked onto the ward. Five of the nuns from Mother Theresa's Order, the Sisters of Charity. They certainly got some looks from the nurses and other patients on the ward!

I'm not a Catholic, I wouldn't consider myself religious. However, I have grown fond of one of the nuns, Sister Terracina.

I guess I should explain how I built a relationship with them. Kind of accidently, I'd started working with them. Mother Theresa had been to the UK and decided that several beds at their convent in South East London should be for people who were dying of AIDS-related illnesses. The HIV organizations in London hadn't really engaged with the nuns, and I was introduced to them by a friend who thought I may be able to help. I didn't have much success with helping them carry out Mother Theresa's wish, but I did strike up a relationship with them. I would visit them at the convent from time to time, and they would sometimes give me books to read. On one visit I was given a copy of *The Prophet* by Kahlil Gibran. I would read the books and then go back and discuss them.

When Sister Terracina found out I was in hospital again, the nuns did something they'd never done before. Five of them jumped into their little car (it was a Mini Metro. I used to call it "the Nun Mobile") and came without warning to see me.

After a time, Sister Terracina asked if they could pray for me. I thought it kind and said of course. They stood around my bed and prayed and left shortly afterwards. I didn't really know what to make of the experience, but I felt loved and cared for. They are very special people.

SEVERAL MONTHS LATER...

[Diary] Wednesday 28th June, 1995
I'm back in hospital. Strangely enough, I'm in the same bed, on the same bay as I was before. I had a temperature of 39.5 degrees Celsius last night. I've also been having chest pains. They started about a week ago. My first thought was that it may have been the return of PCP, an AIDS-related pneumonia that I had last year, but I had only recently had prophylaxis treatment to prevent me from getting it, and I'd eliminated it from the list of potential illnesses in the Pandora's Box that is AIDS. The pain had gotten worse – in fact, I'd never known pain quite like this. It felt as though my lungs were sticking to my chest. I know, Dear Diary, that doesn't make sense at all, but I'm not sure how else to describe it.

Some friends and I have planned to go to a nightclub that operates a strict 1970s theme. I bought my outfit last week. I was really looking forward to going. I had taken some heavy-duty painkillers that I had found in the medicine box, left-overs from some other painful AIDS-related event. I tried not to let my condition stop me from enjoying myself and went to the nightclub with my friends. I danced, something quite unusual for me – I'm not a natural dancefloor fiend. Maybe enjoying whatever was left, because I knew deep down something wasn't right.

ONE MONTH LATER...

[Diary] Wednesday 26th July, 1995

I went to the clinic for a routine check-up. The doctor asked how I was and I told him I was felt I was recovering slowly from my recent infection. He left the room momentarily and came back with my medical notes. He pointed out that a sticker had been placed on the cover. It was a big red capital letter "T". He explained that was because I'd been on the ward when TB had been transmitted to others – it was nothing to worry about, but was just so they could keep an eye on me. The doctor told me they believed I had escaped infection.

I feel some relief at this. It had come to mind, hearing that others who'd been there at the same time had been isolated, that I too may be infected. The doctor has told me, however, that I'm probably alright and not to worry. Although I hadn't tried to think about it too much, it had bothered me on some level, and I walked out of the clinic feeling some relief.

[Diary] Thursday 27th July, 1995

Today, I'm finishing my first book (Positive Carers: The Rights and Responsibilities of HIV-Positive Healthcare Workers); it's nearly done and I'm looking forward to it being published. The last thing I wrote was the Acknowledgments page, and I feel a real sense of achievement for having gotten this far. As I wrote the final page, three years of hard work were coming to an end, and I got tearful. I think it was because I'm happy more than anything else.

As I wrote, the telephone rang. My partner, Tony, told me that the hospital was trying to get hold of me urgently. I started to feel a strange sense of dread. And then he told me. The doctors thought that I might have MDR-TB.

I telephoned my doctor straight away. He told me that they'd grown something called 'acid-fast bacilli' (AFB) from the induced sputum sample that I'd given back the month before. This meant nothing to me. He says that I may have TB and needed to go to the hospital urgently. I went cold. I didn't think it even existed anymore.

I put the phone down. Although I'd been calm on the phone with the doctor, I felt panic welling up inside me. I told the people in the office what I'd been told. The situation was so odd. No one knew what to say to me at first. I realised that they too had been at risk; for nearly three months I'd sat there with them. I started to cry. I felt so guilty. TB – but how? It was so... Victorian. Had I known that I might've been putting people at risk, I would never have gone back to work.

By the time I'd packed away my things, Tony had arrived in the car to take me to the hospital. I didn't know what to say. I felt like I was watching myself through a window. Someone hugged me, I don't know who. I wasn't thinking, but I really needed that hug. Being rejected would have devastated me.

Tony took me home first so that I could grab a few things and make a few phone calls. I don't have any contact with my family; on hearing I was HIV-positive my father, believing that being gay was a choice, told me that I'd made my bed and now I must lie in it. Tony was the closest thing I had to family.

We made our way in the car to the hospital and,

once on the ward, I was put into a side room on my own. I waited for a couple of hours; the whole situation felt distant, as though it wasn't happening to me. Occasionally a nurse would poke her head around the door to see if I was okay. I felt so guilty, but I didn't know why. I felt like I'd done something wrong.

Eventually my doctor came in and tried to explain to me what was happening. It had been decided that I would be placed in a negative-pressure isolation room, and this was being prepared for me as we spoke. The doctor told me that, basically, this is a specially-designed room where air pressure is lower than outside so infection can't get out.

The doctor tried to get across the gravity of the situation, but said I should be okay. I found this confusing: they suspected that I had TB and I was being put into isolation as a precaution while they did further tests. I felt they knew that they had to do something positive quickly, but they seemed as surprised as me. The doctor compared my situation to what had happened in America in the recent past, and kept stressing the need to halt any potential epidemic. An *epidemic*? What is happening?!

What have I become, a time bomb ticking away?

What about the person who had infected me? In the meantime, they've asked me to write a list of everyone I've been in contact with since April 14th, 1995. How could I do this? I'd been to restaurants, on the subway – my head started to whirl. Were things that bad? Again, I felt as though I was watching all of this on TV. I wanted it to stop, but I knew it wouldn't. It was like having a nightmare that I couldn't wake up from.

I made my own way to the ward where I was to spend my time in isolation while they tried definitively to diagnose me with TB. As we walked, Tony joked that the nurses may be waiting there with a broomstick, or an electric cattle prod to make sure I didn't come too close. I couldn't help but laugh.

I was led down the corridor to the room. The door closed behind me and I sat down on the bed. They say it's 'isolation'. What does this mean? Can I see anybody? Too many questions and too few answers. How could my day have turned out like this? This morning, I was happy; I'd finished my book. Now they've locked me up and I may be about to become very sick, perhaps even die. I can't write anymore...

LATER...

[Diary] Thursday 27th July, 1995 (continued)

The walls of the isolation room are pink, and a picture of a dove is hung opposite the bed. When I arrived in the room it had no curtains. It's standard infection-control procedure to remove them when someone vacates a room. I was told that a new set would arrive today, but they haven't yet. I wondered if they would? How do I feel? I don't really know. Doctors are so used to this sort of thing, but I'm not. I need it explained to me, but it's difficult to take on board what they're saying. My world has turned upside down on a dime.

They've started me on intravenous treatment but my vein collapsed soon after they started the drug, and nothing's going through it. It just pools in the flesh. A doctor removed the needle and has put in another one. They've told me the bacteria they found in my sample (AFB) is now being tested for DNA evidence of TB. It's going to take a few days to get a result. More waiting.

I'm starting to feel a bit hemmed in. They have told me I can't leave the room until I'm told I can. I feel a like I've been a naughty boy. This must be a punishment...

My first meal arrived, and I remembered how much I hated hospital food. I'm a good cook and really miss great food. Each time I've been in hospital in the past I seem to have lost weight! On previous occasions I have gotten friends to bring 'edible' food in for me. They say I'm fussy, and that hospital food is good for me. I say, "Then you eat it!"

When my friends finally arrived they were wearing masks, plastic aprons and gloves. It felt strange having people I know wrapped up in this way. It made me feel tearful and guilty again. They felt initially awkward with the masks on. I missed seeing their faces as we talked. It is funny how much we read into a face: they must be observed in the context of some other expression. A smile, perhaps?

[Diary] Friday 28th July, 1995

I'm being given anti-TB treatment as a precaution while they do further tests to confirm the diagnosis. The needle they put in my arm to give me intravenous medication felt raw this morning. Again, the vein collapsed and now nothing will go through it. The thought of a vein collapsing makes me shudder. (They removed the needle and replaced it later in the day and the IV TB therapy was recommenced.)

[Diary] Saturday 29th July, 1995

The days seem to be blending into each other and I'm finding it difficult to tell on which day events are happening. I am so bored. I've decided to dedicate more time to my diary so that I can really keep track of what's going on. At least I have something to occupy my mind.

I've noticed that my dreams are becoming confused with reality. The diary may at least help me define what was real and what wasn't. I've also asked Tony to bring my watch in so that I had some concept of time. The clean curtains have arrived, and I'm making the effort to open them during the day and close them at night in the hope that they may help me distinguish one from the other. I'm not sure what's real anymore. I know I have a temperature, and I'd wake up thinking I'd been outside, but I knew that wasn't possible. I think this is because of the medication I'm being given. It feels very strong. I don't feel right at all. I'm trying to watch scheduled TV programmes, such as the news – I need to keep a grip of what is reality. My head is a dangerous neighborhood to be in alone.

[Diary] Sunday 30ᵗʰ July, 1995

I still don't have any news on the further tests they're performing on my sputum sample. I find this quite annoying. The nurse keeps telling me that the results will come tomorrow, but tomorrow never seems to come. I know they're busy, but because I'm in isolation, it's all I must think about. Each sample I've given for a basic smear test for TB bacteria has come back negative. This surely must be good news, right? I may still have TB, but hopefully I'm not infectious. They've told me that if things stay like this, and if I don't have a fever, I can go home. If I do develop a temperature or if a test comes back positive, I'd have to stay. If the latter were the case, I would have to produce three negative smear samples, with no temperature, for at least a week before I could go. It feels like a bizarre game. I'm glad I'm writing all of this down, as there's a lot to understand.

[Diary] Monday 31ˢᵗ July, 1995

I'm climbing the fucking walls. I've lost a lot of weight; my muscles are starting to waste as I can't exercise in such a small room. I have some vertigo from one of the drugs I'm being given and diarrhea from another. At least I haven't had a temperature and my tests have been negative for the week. But no one will commit to saying that I do not have MDR-TB.

I hate the colour pink.

[Diary] Wednesday 2nd August, 1995

I woke this morning having had one of the worst night's sleep ever. It's odd – I usually sleep pretty well. I lay awake most of the time trying to piece together what was happening to me. A note had been placed on my bedside table written by my doctor. It said that "guidelines were not written in stone", and that I had given negative smear tests for a week, and that this meant I may be able to go home. It appeared I wasn't infectious. I was so happy that I was almost certainly not a danger to others: even if I had TB, it didn't seem to be active.

Eventually a junior doctor came to see me and told me I could go home, although I would have to wait for the TB drugs they were giving me as a precautionary measure. Did that mean I could walk out of the room right then? She paused for a moment – she couldn't see why not.

She left the room and I stood there for a

moment, frozen, almost as if I didn't want to leave. I'd become used to the close confines of isolation. Then I turned and, holding up the pyjama bottoms that were now far too big for me, I ran out the door...

The heat hit me; I hadn't realised that everyone else was suffering a heat wave. My room had been air-conditioned and the temperature hadn't changed much. For the first time in a week I made my own cup of tea. Cups of tea were virtually the only thing that I asked for when I pressed the red call button for the nurses. I sat in the day room with other people. How amazing to be around people again. However, not all my news was good news.

One of the nurses needed to give me some information before I left. He came into the room where I was celebrating my freedom, and broke news to me that was going to change my situation dramatically.

I couldn't believe what I was being told. As a precaution, I was to stay away from all people I knew to be HIV-positive for at least two months, at which time the situation would be re-evaluated. I was devastated; most of my friends were from the HIV organization where I worked, and Tony was also

HIV-positive. I remonstrated with him, then was told that, apparently, I was lucky someone had suggested I couldn't mix with other people who were HIV-positive for two years! I was so desperate to spend time with people I knew after being alone, but I couldn't. Did I really have to stay at home for two months and not see *anyone*? It felt like I was going from isolation in hospital to isolation at home.

I went back to the room and collected the bits and pieces that I'd collected over the week and loaded them into my rucksack. Something wasn't right. I decided to go and speak to the Ward Sister. Presumably I was being discharged because I was non-infectious, right? Why must I stay away from people, those who cared about me, my network? I ended up having a row with her. When she couldn't answer my questions, she told me they were letting me out "because I wanted to go". I told her in no uncertain terms that this was complete rubbish. If they were letting me go purely because I wanted to, then this was irresponsible of them. At this, she replied, "Well, we can always put you back into isolation again." I asked her if I could quote her on that... she rolled her eyes. Terrified, I got out of there as quickly as possible. Outside the hospital main entrance I sat on the floor, surrounded by the belongings from my room, and cried. I was so relieved to be out and (presumably) not infectious, but at the same time devastated at not being able to see my friends at this trying time. I was prepared, however, to do whatever they wanted, for fear that they would take me prisoner.

[NOTE]

Over the next few weeks I was started on TB medication as a precautionary measure. I questioned the doctor about the situation. Unable to answer my questions, he, like the Ward Sister, suggested they could always put me back in isolation again. Too frightened to ask any more questions that no one seemed to be able to answer, and of the threat of being locked up again, for the time being I stopped asking them.

PART 2 - CURE

"Risk! Risk anything! Care no more for the opinions of others, for those voices. Do the hardest thing on earth for you. Act for yourself. Face the truth."

The Letters of Katherine Mansfield

[Celia Hall, writing in the *The Independent*] Thursday 17th August, 1995

"A London hospital has changed its procedures following an outbreak of Multidrug-resistant tuberculosis in which one patient may have infected four others on an AIDS ward.

More than 52 contacts of the patients involved have been identified, and public health doctors in 12 local authorities across the United Kingdom are now offering them a TB test. It is believed to be the first UK outbreak of the serious strain of TB, and public health officials are taking it "extremely seriously".

The first patient, who had HIV and has since died, was isolated as soon as the diagnosis was made but he produced sputum samples on an open six-bed ward which he shared with five other patients over two days...

Tuberculosis is passed on from one person to another through airborne droplets expelled in coughing or sneezing. This type of TB, known as MDR-TB, has caused serious problems in New York among the HIV and drug-injecting populations. It is identified as TB which is resistant to at least two of the "first-line" TB drugs, isoniazid and rifampicin."

[Diary] Friday 4th August, 1995

This morning the district nurse came to see me. The doctors have put me on a programme called Direct Observed Therapy, or DOT for short. This means that I must be watched taking my medication twice a day. I feel a bit like a naughty boy. Firstly, locked up in my room and told to stay there until I can come out, and now 'Nana' says that good boys must take their medicine.

I'm in a foul mood... One thing's for sure, the Ward Sister won't be rolling her eyes when she finds out that my question about quoting her on locking me up again was genuine. Or not. I have one of two choices... to give up or fight. I've chosen the latter. I'll do whatever it takes, whatever the consequences. Let's see what I can do, if only in the nature of an experiment. I have nothing to lose now.

[Diary] Wednesday 9th August, 1995

The telephone rang this morning. It was Professor Robert Pratt, author of *HIV and AIDS: A Strategy for Nursing Care*. He's my old Vice-Principle from when I was at the School of Nursing. His record with his book is impressive. It's been printed in nine different languages and it's in its fourth edition now. I can only dream of such writing success. We agreed that we would meet at Pimlico subway station near where I live. Robert has been to my house before. He read some of my stuff when I was writing *Positive Carers* and was very encouraging. I'm having to meet him, though, as he can't quite remember where I live.

I walked down to the subway. The district nurse had not yet been to give me my injection, and I was worried that she might come while I was out. She may report me if I'm not compliant with instructions. I'd only waited by the escalators a short time when I saw Robert rising with a bunch of other people from the depths of the station.

Robert and I walked up the road towards my flat. We'd discussed on the phone about writing an article for *Nursing Times*, to be published the week after as their major news story. We got to my flat, Robert got his laptop out and the work began. We used my diary and notes that I'd taken while in hospital as a reference. He'd seen them the previous night after I'd faxed them to him. He says he likes my style of writing.

He started to type, and quizzed me thoroughly about what happened on the ward. While we did this, we saw a powerful story emerging. My diary concentrated on how my diagnosis affected me and how I believed my civil liberties had been violated. It clearly started to emerge from the discussion that I was in this situation because I'd been infected in the first place.

How? Because the very people who'd placed me on the medication with their terrible side effects, also placed the restrictions on me not to go near anyone who was thought to be HIV-positive because there may be an infection risk, had also carried out several induced sputum tests on another patient on the open ward. There is a high probability that poor infection control led to the mess that I find myself in.

After writing the article with Robert, he faxed it to *Nursing Times*.

Later, I spoke to the journalist dealing with the article. He told me that there were going to be three parts to it. My piece, Robert's piece and a bit by the journalist himself. It was to be their main feature. I was feeling the effects of the medication I am taking and felt, frankly, a bit mad.

I called Robert and let him know that *Nursing Times* really liked the article. He told me that a photographer had been and had taken pictures of him and his secretary. He got her to wear a facemask, and joked he would make her a star.

[Diary] Thursday 10th August, 1995

I cried again last night. I feel so confused. I know it's the medication and there's a distinct feeling that I'm going to have to fight a battle. Sometimes I feel so strong and other times so weak. Crying is something that I've never been very good at, but in the last few weeks I've found it's relieved some of the tension I've felt.

I'm trying to focus on the fact that it is the

medication that's making me feel this way. It's strong and makes me feel woozy, but I know I must take it. I've decided to change where I receive care. I have absolutely no faith whatsoever in the hospital where I may have contracted this terrible disease. I got ready to go to St Mary's hospital in Paddington, London. I caught a cab and was feeling slightly hot, and I couldn't make up my mind if it was because it was a hot day, was just because I was nervous or if I genuinely had a temperature. The latter worried me more; would this mean that if the doctor at St Mary's saw I had even a slight temperature they, too, would lock me away?

I met my new doctor for the first time. I told him my story, and he busily made notes as I related to him what had happened as best as I could understand. I'd prepared a letter the night before, stating that I was transferring my care to him. I was given a couple of sample containers and we arranged that I'd come back again the next day. I took a cab home.

[Diary] Friday 11th August, 1995
I still haven't gotten used to the district nurse coming so early to watch me take my medication. I've never

been an early riser. She arrived about 9.30am. Her name's Valerie: I quite like her because she talks and has tea with me. I want to talk to her about the side effects I'm having, but I don't quite know how. The drugs seem to affect my way of thinking, as well as the more physical side effects.

I'm still sore from the injections I've had over the past four days. We had been alternating where they went: right buttock one day, left the next. They're deep injections and I've never been very good with needles. The fact remains that I don't know which way to sit because my bottom is so sore. My legs feel like lead and it's becoming difficult to move about.

After Valerie left, my friend took me back to the hospital so I could hand in some more sputum samples, as we had arranged yesterday. I didn't have a cough and it was difficult to bring anything up. A few slaps on the back seemed to get the ball rolling. I like the phrase "cough in a pot"; it reminds me of "cat in the hat"!

I hoped, as I walked upstairs to the clinic, that I'd coughed up enough. The nurses asked me how I was feeling. I told them all right, barring the side effects of the medication. They took some blood, and that was it. Time to go. My legs feel so stiff. I think it might be because the streptomycin is put into the muscle, but I'm not sure. There's so much I am unsure about, in fact...

I'm amazed that I got home without collapsing. I can only assume this was because of the injections and the other drugs I'm taking. I should really ask. I need to know these things.

When I got home I lay down on my bed. I put on a healing tape. My partner absolutely hates it! He says it's New Age crap. Whatever he may think, it sort of half-worked. The digital clock flicked over. It was 5.30 in the afternoon. I lay back into the four pillows I had stacked up and poured on some lavender oil. My back feels so knotted up, and all I can do is toss and turn restlessly. I start to relax after a while and my legs began to feel slightly better.

[Diary] Saturday 12th August, 1995

The doorbell rang about 10am. It was the district nurse again. I'd slept quite well that night. I must have been tired, and when I got up to answer the door I was surprised to see how late it was. I took my pills and had my injection. I was too tired to talk. I wanted to ask about side effects again, but I didn't feel up to it.

Later I sat there alone. The effects of the tablets had really taken hold by now. I moved off the sofa onto the floor and crawled to my bedroom and onto the bed. The smooth tones from my New Age tape rang out, and I was flinging lavender oil around the room. It mixed with the smell of my burning cigarette, from which I was taking a deep draw. Stab. A pain flared in my chest. It got worse. My throat felt dry, I started to cough. Something wasn't right, and it wasn't just the side effects I was feeling. I thought back to the samples I'd given to the hospital: will they want to isolate me again if they find out how I'm starting to feel? My head feels like a merry-go-round.

I'm so frightened every time there's a knock on the door, or if the phone rings. If a cop car comes down the street, I wonder if they're coming for me. It's the deranging effects of this medication: I know it alters my thoughts, but it still feels real. I must be paranoid! I don't know what's real anymore. I feel like I'm living with the daily prospect of being locked up, like some sort of fugitive. The nearest thing to this that I have ever been through is being sent to my room as a child, only this isn't a child's game. It is all far too adult.

I lit another cigarette and felt that pain in my chest again. It was quite constant, and I wondered if this was a side effect or the disease they were trying to prevent. I lay there for what must have been hours. Then the doorbell: it was about 6pm. It was the district nurse. She came in, watched me take my pills and left.

I was alone again. The pain was still there. I hadn't told her about it. I hoped it would go away. I wanted it to go away. I didn't have a temperature, but the pain was familiar. By 8.30pm I was very worried. The pain hadn't gone and now I had a temperature. I wasn't coughing anything up. Perhaps I was over-reacting?

I have read in my *Complete Home Medical Encyclopedia of Symptoms* by Dr Sigmund Stephen Miller that TB can "occur insidiously, with a slow loss of weight and gradual insidious fatigue and then explode into what is often chillingly called 'galloping consumption'. In a short space of time the patient becomes emaciated, his skin turns greyish, he develops a cough with bloody sputum and almost every night drenches his bed with sweat. Before the advent of new drugs, 'galloping consumption' would kill in a matter of weeks."

I could almost hear the voice of Hammer Horror actor Vincent Price in my head as I read the description. I even tried reading the section out loud in his voice. It wasn't long before I fell about in fits of laughter. Perhaps I *am* going mad? Then the fear again. I was terrified 'it' was going to get me. Was I going to be chucking up gallons of frothy blood, and then explode into 'galloping consumption', just like the book said? Up until now I haven't really suffered from any actual symptoms of the disease as described by the book. My main problems are the psychological ones of dealing with what might happen to me, and the effects of the medication on my head. They had progressed from bad to worse. Things are so uncertain. I will try not to be frightened tonight as I go to bed. Perhaps by morning it will have passed?

[Diary] Sunday 13th August, 1995

The noise of the doorbell blended into my dreaming. I woke with a start when, for a second time, the district nurse pushed the button: longer this time. I struggled out of bed. I wasn't feeling too good this morning. I'd only managed to get about four hours sleep: it wasn't a constant sleep, but it was all I could grab in between the hours of worry.

The district nurse commented on how I looked. I told her that I never looked my best when I woke up. (Judging by the look of her, she probably didn't either, I thought.) I wasn't in the mood this morning. A handful of pills and an injection later, and she was gone into the ether again.

I smoked the last cigarette in the packet. I'm smoking more than I usually do these days. About 40 a day. Still, this is better than when I was in the isolation room, when I was smoking about 60 a day. I had put some of the pain I felt in my chest down to my excessive smoking. Today, my chest's feeling better, I'm not coughing and I haven't got a temperature. This is something to be glad about. I don't think they'll isolate me again if I don't have any of these symptoms.

I realised that my appointment to find out my sputum results was scheduled for about 5pm the next day. Originally, it was going to be at 2.30pm, but they changed their minds. Was this in anticipation of me being infectious, and them not wanting me to sit in the waiting room with lots of other people? Were they ready to admit me the next day? Was this my last day of freedom? I am feeling totally paranoid.

I must try to keep things in perspective, underneath the weight of the medication. I must focus on the day or even the moment, and just to try and keep my sanity. I asked myself: "Am I infected or not?"; "Am I a danger to other people?". These are difficult questions to answer, especially when so many of the factors involved are unknown.

I feel as though I'm swinging between feeling quite well and feeling ill. My legs still feel like lead; sometimes I wake up and feel paralysed for a few minutes. It's not a feeling I enjoy. I used to sleep well, but now it's a chore to get through the night. Even my stupid New Age tape and lavender oil don't work, things I used to swear by. Perhaps it *is* all New Age crap after all, as my friends tell me?

The fear of dying comes and goes. The thought that I may be dead in a few months and die alone in some clinical isolation unit away from those I love fills me with such fear. I fantasize. If I was dead, at least I wouldn't be frightened anymore.

I went to bed at about 10pm, which is quite early for me – something didn't feel right. When I woke up I judged it to be about 4.30am. I thought I'd been asleep for a while. To my surprise, the clock showed

11.30pm.

The pain in my chest had gotten worse and I was having difficulty stopping myself from coughing. I took another painkiller and then took my temperature. I knew I had one, I just didn't know how high.

After a minute or so I took the thermometer out of my mouth and twiddled it around to read it: 38.5 degrees Celsius. I knew what I had to do, and telephoned the hospital. I couldn't wait for my appointment at 5pm to get my result. My body was already telling me what it would be.

I arrived at the hospital and went to the Casualty department. I sort of 'floated around' when I arrived. I wasn't sure what to do or what they were going to do to me. Eventually I was put in a room away from everyone else. I sat on the couch which had no cover, just naked plastic. I would have liked to have lain down, but the grease stains left by the hair of the last occupant put me off. An hour and a half later and still no one had come. I looked to the wall for a nurse call button, there wasn't one. I sat cross-legged on the couch.

Eventually, a nurse came in and gave me a mask, which she asked me to wear, and then indicated for me to follow her. I carried my own bag, which seemed to get heavier and heavier while she walked a good 4 metres ahead of me. I was feeling so bad. By the time we reached the ward, the gap had grown to about 10 metres due to my exhaustion. She told me to stand outside the ward and left me by the door.

I was greeted by another nurse, who seemed more pleasant, and she showed me to my room. It wasn't a negative-pressure room.

Once I was in, another nurse came in wearing one of the masks. She had brought some tea and toast with her. She told me that the doctor would be in to see me soon and that I'd be moved out of the room to a real negative-pressure room... when the builders had finished working on it! She left, and I was alone again, my head propped up by a couple of thin pillows – with clean pillow cases, thank God.

Eventually the doctor came. He was obviously tired from having worked all weekend. He told me that the doctors and nurses in Casualty had been worried about me being there. The radiographers also didn't feel sure about me attending the X-ray department because of possible infection. I asked him questions about my potential problems: he told me that he didn't have any answers, as he had only come to check me in. I asked him how he felt about being in the same room with me. He said he was apprehensive. I thanked him for our chat: it had been a good half-hour long.

I must try to let go. There is only so much I can do, and the situation is out of my control. I must try to sleep. I've taken a sleeping tablet and it's starting to work.

[Diary] Monday 14th August, 1995

Another cup of tea and a couple of slices of toast greeted me, but before I could eat anything another nurse had come in to take my temperature. It was 38.2 degrees Celsius, quite high for me in the morning. It was usually high at night. I had my breakfast and after that another cigarette in anticipation of the Consultant coming around to see me.

I'd fallen asleep by the time he arrived. My neck was wet from sweating, and when I woke I found I'd soaked my pillow. He examined me thoroughly while his entourage watched: he told me that he wasn't convinced this episode was down to TB. The nurse took the two samples of the sputum I had produced that morning, and the Consultant *et al* left the room. I then rediscovered the delights of daytime TV…

It's so bloody hot in here, and I can't open the window – it's been nailed down. I'm not allowed to have a fan as it would affect the pressure in the room and blow any tubercle bacilli out through the door when people came in.

There's a fly in my room, and it will never get out.

[Diary] Tuesday 15th August, 1995

I woke in the still, airless room. I had my usual cup of tea and a cigarette. The weatherman says it's going to be hot again today. I'm at Day 19 and still no news. I don't know whether I have this disease or not. I walked over to the window to get my urine bottle, and next to it lay the fly. Dead.

A senior Radiographer came crashing through the door with a machine resembling a big, white robot. She told me she was the only one who was prepared to come. The other Radiologists had declined. I felt hurt by this. Still, she stayed for about 10 minutes and chatted.

I'm so busy wondering what's going to happen next, I'm finding it difficult to live within the moment. Still, perhaps in here the moment is not the best thing to think about? It's so dismal. I think back to how that one phone call came out of the blue in July. My whole life was totalled in a few seconds. Perhaps that's why I'm so scared of what will happen next, because you just don't know what's around the corner. I guess none of us does.

I could hear and see a group of doctors through the slatted glass window in the door. They talked for a few seconds before they came in. I was getting impatient: they hadn't been able to get any test results. I showed them my contempt by being abrupt and rude when they entered. I had a good rant about it, but the doctor interrupted me: they had got my test results back that morning. These confirmed that I had MDR-TB.

[Diary] Wednesday 16th August, 1995

The newspaper vendor came about 11am, a nurse ran in; "He's got a *Nursing Times*; quick, give me some money!" I gave her some and a few seconds later she ran back with a copy of the magazine.

I nervously flicked through the pages, and there, a picture of me jumped off the pages. I was re-reading the article I'd written with Robert, when who should walk through the door but Robert himself! He wasn't wearing a mask like everyone else who came into my room did. He agreed with me that it had been edited quite a bit, but it still worked. I was most pleased that I was able to quote the Ward Sister who'd said that they could always lock me up again. I guess she isn't rolling her eyes now! Robert and I chatted about things in general and before he went he left a rolled-up carrier bag with five packets of cigarettes inside.

I sat alone cross-legged on my bed. It was 32 degrees Celsius outside. The dirty brickwork of the enclosed square of buildings outside my window looked beautiful. How I'd have loved to be out there!

Later that night, I was moved to my new room that the builders had finished. It was more bearable than the room I had; they'd knocked down a wall and I now had a bathroom. It was quite large, as it had been a communal bathroom before. The shower didn't seem capable of any real pressure – it was reminiscent of an old man with a prostate problem urinating! However, I'm grateful for the small amount of cold water the shower provides – it doesn't do hot! One of the other benefits of the bathroom is that it's quite cool and offers some respite from the heat of the main room – it doesn't have much of a window other than a small one over the toilet. I could see me spending a lot of time in the bathroom hiding from the heat.

[Diary] Friday 18th August, 1995

I woke, tossing and turning, still drowsy from the previous night's sleeping tablet, to a small pile of mail by my bed. I lay drenched in sweat. I was cold, but one of the letters received was colder. It chilled my blood.

[Letter] Friday 18th August, 1995

Paul,

Truly and sincerely sorry to hear that you have Multidrug-resistant tuberculosis. I wouldn't wish that affliction on a dog or a pig – truly!

However, I must say that you have brought it on yourself by choosing to adopt a 'queer' lifestyle.

Have you ever considered emigrating to Zimbabwe where you will be warmly welcomed by

President Robert Mugabwe as an asset to his economy? I believe he is… encouraging queers and lesbos to migrate there.

You are quoted as saying that you are angry at being infected with Multidrug-resistant tuberculosis. Well, Paul, let me tell you that millions of us long-suffering 'straights' are angry too. Angry that faggots like you have the affrontery to complain at all the treatment you are receiving; when you have self-inflicted the illness due to your disgusting lifestyle. You are bleeding the National Health coffers dry. This money would be better spent in the third world eliminating leprosy, for example. People like you are viral ticking time bombs, harboring Multidrug-resistant tuberculosis and God alone knows what else. You are not fit to live in civilized society. Perhaps Zimbabwe is the place for you after all."

Fed-Up Straight, Rochester

[Diary] Friday 18th August, 1995 (continued)

The letter had been posted in a brown envelope and typed with an old-fashioned typewriter. It had the feeling of a poison pen letter; short of cutting out the individual letters from the daily newspaper and gluing them together, this was the next best thing. For the first time, I felt comfort and safety within the four walls of the isolation room.

I've received many letters while in my prison. I don't know who sent most of them. They're mainly from people who had heard about what had happened through the newspapers or who picked up the story from the *Nursing Times*. None of them has been like the one I received this morning.

I needed to wake up and try and get dry. I pressed the call button on the keypad that rested beside me in the wet sheets. When I took a close look at the button it made me smile. There's a 'stick-woman' picture of a nurse, wearing a pointy, triangular dress, and in her hand there's a tray with a cup on it. A couple of nurses, anonymous in their masks, came in. They didn't knock. As they peeled the sheets away from the vinyl mattress, I busied myself in the shower, if that's what you could call it. Little seemed to work properly in the room. There was *never* any hot water. I can tell you that it is quite a shock to the system when you've been consumed by fever all night and face a cold shower. At least I could get clean. I hadn't been able to bring myself to stand there under the cold mid-stream of the shower for the previous few days. Nor had I shaved. I looked scruffy.

After I cleaned up, I dried myself down with the rough towel marked 'hospital property'. The room was heating up again. It had been a glorious summer up until that point, and I had experienced none of it. I thought of the people on beaches and walking in the woods, having barbeques and garden parties. My world doesn't extend beyond the metal bars at my window, its frame firmly nailed down, a slight gap between sealed with rubber sealant. Like the shower, the air-conditioning unit wasn't working properly either. It was going to be like a sweathouse again. Opening the window isn't an option. Having a fan isn't, either. I'm not being denied these 'luxuries' out of spite. It's a necessity, they say. To risk altering the air pressure in the room could potentially lead to infectious TB bacteria being blown out of the door into the rest of the hospital. Others could possibly be infected with the terrible disease that I now harbor in my lungs.

The nurses had left a surgical gown on the bottom of the newly-made bed. Today was going to be different to the others. I was going to be allowed to take a walk. To nowhere more interesting than another room in the hospital. Once you've seen a few they all begin to look a bit the same. Magnolia paint – "prison white with a hint of institution". It was, however, going to be a chance to breathe some different air. I'm looking forward to it. What I'm not looking forward to is the camera being passed down into my lungs.

I was to be sedated during the procedure, called a bronchoscopy. I've never had this procedure before, and I'm terrified. Will it feel like I'm drowning when they pass the camera into my lungs?

A few hours have passed since I last wrote, and although it's not as hot as yesterday, it's still very warm in the room. I haven't been able to eat or drink anything since I had breakfast this morning. I'm feeling very dehydrated. At 4pm and they took me down to perform the procedure. It was great just to feel and smell the new air as I walked. It felt different, moist, unlike the air in my room.

When the staff saw me, I could hear them saying: "He's coming, he's coming," and saw them frantically putting on their masks. Sister had briefed me the day before on what the procedure would involve. This time, she wasn't wearing her uniform, but was in an outfit that resembled a space suit in a bad 1950s' 'B' movie, and so was my doctor. Both had special respiratory equipment. Sister then grabbed my shoulders and, pushing from behind, frogmarched me to the bronchoscopy suite. I lay on the couch, as they asked, and co-operated with their other requests. Sister wasn't going to take any nonsense from me today! I certainly wasn't going to mess with her. She was bigger than me and I didn't want to wrestle with her in my condition. I quickly asked whatever runs the Universe to keep me safe.

The first injection was to dry any secretions, then an injection of the sedative. I looked at the wall. It didn't feel as though it was working. Please let it work, I don't want to remember. I thought about the panic when I had arrived. "He's coming, he's coming." My world turned to darkness and I didn't care.

[Letter] Friday 18th August, 1995

Dear Paul,

Thanks for your letter. Who got gold stars at school from teacher for such beautiful handwriting?

Forgive me from for saying this, but you do

yourself an injustice. It is me that gains strength from you. You are the fighter. You are facing battles that I can only begin to imagine. Some of them you will win, some of them you will lose. Remember, Paul, whatever happens you will come out as a winner because you stood and fought – you didn't give up even when you wanted to. If a little of your fighting spirit can be passed onto others, as it will be, you will have done more good than you can possibly imagine.

It is only fairly recently that I admitted I was gay. I think most people decide they are gay, get on with it and then decide to come out. I am doing it all at once and it is a bit of a roller coaster in just about every way I can imagine. (I need a thesaurus – I've used the word 'imagine' three times already!)

You said that your biggest fear was being rejected by the gay community. A community which rejects its own doesn't have a right to exist – not in my book, anyway. I have to confess to be being totally confused at the moment. One side to the community is 'the scene' which seems so shallow and inconsequential and then on the other you have all these guys looking out for each other, supporting one another as friends and lovers fall to AIDS. I *guess if I try to make sense of it all, I shall end up a bit schizo!*

Life is a peculiar thing – strength comes from unexpected sources when you are not expecting it. A few months ago, I bought a book Becoming a Man – Half a Life's Story *by Paul Monette. It was about his experience of spending years in the closet and finally coming out. I found it incredibly inspirational (despite him being American!). I followed this up with a book he wrote as a series of essays as he faced his battle with AIDS. A book (entitled* Last Watch of Night*) has never made me cry before, but the following had me in floods:*

"For me it began in a small town in Massachusetts forty years ago – a sickness of the soul about being different. And nothing more important, not breath itself, than the need to keep it a secret. The stillborn journey of my life took off at the last, the moment I opened the closet door. To know how dank a place you come from into the light of self-acceptance – it is to enact a sort of survivorship that leaves a trail for those who come after you. But you don't carry that bit with you the rest of your life – wounded as he is by hate and lies – a shadow companion who needs you to free him."

All the fear that some of us had about being gay summed up in one beautifully eloquent passage. It went a long way to restoring my battered spirit after years of torment and self-deception. My journey has started. I know I will never be alone because of guys like you, Paul. The indominatable spirit that permeates the 'tribe' (as Paul Monette calls us) can never, ever be taken away from us.

I would love for us to correspond, whether you want to 'chat' via our letters or use me as a verbal 'punch-bag'. I don't mind. If you want to rail and rage, then do it! Don't be afraid to ask if you need something – the offer re: books or magazines or whatever still stands. I have a little confession to make. I bought you three bars of chocolate and wolfed one myself. SORRY! Let me know when supplies are dwindling, and I will send you some more. The ultimate SOS message – "Send more chocolate".

Take care Paul,
Best Wishes,
P.H., London N21

[Diary] Friday 18th August, (continued)

I stirred. I was in bed again. My mouth was parched, and I wanted a glass of water. The bronchoscopy was over. I couldn't move, let alone summon the strength to push the nurse's call-button. Eventually I managed to push off the oxygen mask that covered my face. My left nostril was very sore. It felt blocked. Apparently, they carry out the procedure mainly through the nose and not the mouth. They never told me that part. Probably just as well, otherwise I may have tried to wriggle from Sister's firm grasp.

I had some difficulty swallowing for a while, but as the hours went by it got easier. My strength was coming back. I'm so tired.

[Diary] Saturday 19th August, 1995

I want to keep as busy as possible. When I'm busy, death feels further away. I wrote a letter to a little girl who I don't know, who had sent drawing of herself playing with her hula-hoop in the garden. A friend of mine had been baby-sitting and had told her about me being here. I was touched: it was so sweet. I'm going to stick it to my bedside cabinet if I can remember to ask the nurse for some medical tape. They usually have some in their pockets.

There's a new addition to my environment; a yellow bucket full of a strange-smelling solution. One of the nurses bought it in earlier. I'm supposed to put all my dirty dishes and cutlery in this bucket. I think this may be a bit of an over-reaction. My disease is airborne; you can't contract it from cutlery or dishes.

It's 1.45am and I've spent the last hour pondering the fact that [despite] all this struggling and fighting, I'm probably going to die anyway. Why do I bother fighting? I have no quality of life here: I can't even see my partner. I just lie here or sit and look at the wall. Even TV has become difficult; it's not as if I'm even watching it when it's on. My concentration span seems so limited.

I need a reason to live and I can't find one, particularly if I must spend the rest of my life in this room, however short. Writing it down seems to provide some comfort; when I'm writing I'm talking about things that have already happened. When I'm left alone with my head and the fear of the future, I don't want to know what's going to happen next, tomorrow, the day after that, or [think about] my bloody predicted demise.

I'm going through feelings of guilt again, like I've

been bad. I feel as though I'm being punished for something; it makes no logical sense because I've done nothing wrong. However, this is precisely how I feel. I've never been in trouble with the cops, so I've never spent time in a cell. Yet, this is still a prison. Unlike most prisoners who can look forward to the time of their release, I'm told that it's uncertain that I'll ever leave this room. They keep on telling me how important it is for me to keep my head together, but I don't have the information to make decisions about my life anymore, and neither do the doctors, or so it seems.

I'd asked the nurse earlier if I could stop TB treatment, and just be allowed to die. It's getting increasingly difficult for them to be positive about my situation. The chances of my survival seem so small. The nurses come in and ask if I'm "okay"; what can I say? "No"? They don't know what to say to that answer, so I just say, "Yes". I'm not telling the truth. It's a plate-spinning act and they're about to fall. Should I just stop trying?

Fighting to survive is encouraged by other human beings: "That's the spirit," they say. They forget that sometimes this is unrealistic. If I die, will people feel I've let them down?

The criterion for my release is negative-sputum test results. How can I even consider the possibility of being well and getting out of here, when my energies should perhaps be better used to prepare for my death? My doctor tells me I'm the only patient he knows who has had MDR-TB and HIV together. Alive, anyhow. I feel very drained at the end of another day in this room. It's been an eventful day for a Saturday. Weekends are usually very quiet.

[Diary] Sunday 20th August, 1995

I had another night sweat last night, around about 4am. The nurse came in to change my sheets. I got back to sleep, only to be woken very early by the breakfast trolley crashing around and being given a bowl of soggy cereal and tepid milk. I spent most of the day sleeping. In my dreams I escape the room- it's a much preferable state to being awake.

[Diary] Monday 21st August, 1995

I woke up at about 8am. The Ward Manager came into my room and started to talk to me about being moved. No one had told me anything about this! I wasn't aware of any move! Apparently, some builders want to build a proper air conditioning and air filtration unit in the room. I'll have to be moved into another room while they do the works. I'll lose my bathroom and toilet for about three days, as the room that I'm moving to doesn't have them. Back to the world of commodes and pee bottles! I hate them. The good news is that even though I apparently have a serious illness, today I'm feeling very well, it must be said. I haven't even got a temperature.

Later, two strange men came into my room and started measuring things up. No, not a coffin for me. They'd noticed a strange duct in the ceiling that disappeared into the bowels of the building. They spent a lot of time peering into it. Where does it go?, seemed to be the question! More importantly, where exactly was the air I'd been breathing going to? It doesn't even bare thinking about. Fair boggles the mind!

A few visitors came to visit me after lunch. While they were there, a domestic came into my room. She had a mop and a bucket with her. In the bucket was a noxious solution that we could smell as she walked through the door. She dipped the mop in the bucket and started to wash the walls with it! It didn't smell right. I asked what the stuff was. Hycolin Phenolic 2%: it came out of a bottle with a skull and crossbones on the label, and a warning that it was harmful and should only be used in well-ventilated spaces. I asked her to get a nurse right away. My visitors by this time had been affected by the fumes and had to leave to room. I wanted to also but couldn't. I tried to find a pocket of breathable air near the floor. There wasn't any.

The nurse came in. My fury was obvious. Who told the domestic to clean my walls with this stuff!? It's a strong disinfectant used to clean rooms after someone had died!! She couldn't tell me. My eyes started to itch, and my skin and throat were burning. The doctor came in to see me: my windpipe felt tight, but he couldn't hear any wheezing and said that I was okay. I completely lost my temper. No wheezing! I've got TB!! Did he really think it was a good idea to use this stuff on the walls? Was it necessary?? He couldn't (or wouldn't) answer my questions. I was so angry; I suppose in a way it gave me the excuse I needed to release a lot of pent-up anger. I shouted and shouted, and I was frightened I wouldn't stop.

Two nurses came in. I told them that they didn't care about me – it made no difference to them whether I lived or died. How could they understand? Why did they pretend to care? One told me that the things I was saying were hurtful. Well, I said the things I did because I was hurting! This was my air, and they had polluted it. I don't want to breathe. At all.

I tried to sleep this afternoon, but people kept coming in to see me. To be frank, I'm getting sick of all these visitors.

Later a doctor came to see me. Another one. I don't know what he looks like because of the orange masks they wear. I must imagine what the rest of someone's face looks like and try to identify them by their hair or possibly glasses. I decided that he might be quite cute under that orange mask from the mental image I drew of his face. Why not?

A senior nurse came in after the doctor and apologised to me for what had happened with the wall-washing incident. It seems one of the nurses who I shouted at had been very upset by the whole thing. She'd been working long hours for a few days now – today was the last day before some time off. I told the senior nurse that I wanted to apologise to her. I forget that the nurses are finding the whole MDR-TB situation hard to deal with, too. It's completely new to them.

The nurse who I had made cry brought me a cup of tea. I turned down the bizarre TV set, which has a mind of its own. (If you turn it up, it gets uncontrollably louder; if you turn it down, it becomes completely inaudible. Like the hot water, nothing works properly in here.) I apologised, and she accepted immediately.

I know that she and the other nurses have tried to do their best for me. Perhaps "Fed-Up Straight" from Rochester was right – how dare I have the affrontery to complain about the treatment that I'm receiving?

[Postcard] Monday 21st August, 1995
(Sent on Postcard of Gilbert and George's picture *Shitty World* (1994))

Dear Paul,

I don't know you – you don't know me. I have just read an article about you. I cannot begin to imagine how you are feeling. I am not a religious guy – but I feel like lighting a candle for you. I will do it tomorrow, I promise. I wish you a lot of courage – Don't give up even if things look bad presently. Apparently, you like chocolates. I hope you will enjoy the ones that I have sent.

P.S. Fruit is the healthier option.

Best wishes,

A.R., London EC2

[Diary] Tuesday 22nd August, 1995

I lay awake in the half-light. The time was 5am. These days, I usually wake up about this time. I don't seem to be covered for the whole night by the sleeping tablets anymore. Perhaps I'm getting used to the sedation. I don't really remember the last proper night's sleep that I had. I smoked several cigarettes and had a couple of cups of tea.

The feeling of being punished for something that I haven't done has come back. The bucket that was left in my room to put cutlery and dishes has been taken away. Another knee-jerk reaction, and pointless. Is this how people with AIDS were treated in the late '80s when no one understood the disease?

I became agitated this afternoon. I haven't had any psychological support for nine days due to a staff shortage. I think that I now know what's meant by the phrase "climbing the walls". I sat down on the floor beside the fridge on the other side of the room with a cup of tea and my cigarettes, purely to see the room from a different perspective. It seemed to work for a while. If anyone had walked, in they might have thought that I'd gone completely mad. And they might have been right.

LATER...

I was woken by the doctor who'd carried out the bronchoscopy. He had the results. He had found an area in my left lung that appears to have cavities forming. He said it was quite inflamed, which indicated that the TB was more active than he'd originally thought. Bad news.

I want oblivion. Sometimes I feel that I'd like to be sedated all the time. The only thing that scares me is that I might not wake up again.

[Diary] Wednesday 23rd August, 1995
If there is a God, I hate him.

[Diary] Thursday 24th August, 1995
The nurse came in to wake me. The time was 7.45am; I was still tired and would have liked to go on sleeping, but the workmen had come to fit the air filtration unit. I had to pack all my things into carrier

bags, taking gulps of tea to wake myself up at the same time. They say it will be only for a few days.

I've been moved to another room: Room 16. Unlike my last room, it doesn't have a double door. I don't think it's a negative-pressure room, although, judging by the walk, it's the farthest room away from the other patients. I have no shower or toilet here. Once again, it's back to the dreaded commode and the urine bottle, and strip- washing at the sink. I won't be able to have a shower for three or four days. There's very little dignity in all of this. I had come to be grateful for the dribble of cold water from the shower, and for having a toilet of my own. One positive point: I get a different perspective of the world, and the chance to breath some different air. My idea of a treat these days!

However, I'm confused enough without being constantly moved around. In addition, the team of nurses looking after me will change. I'd managed to develop some sort of rapport with the other nurses, though it was a bit strained at times. Now I'll have to start again. More new faces – and more new names. All wearing masks with only the eyes visible, so not really new faces at all. It's amazing how much we read into facial expressions. So much is communicated with a smile. No one smiles at me anymore – and if they do I don't get to see it.

I've received no psychological support since I've been here. I've tried my best to manage but sometimes I really lose it and must take diazepam to calm myself. I don't like mind-altering substances. I want to be in control, even if it's only the small things.

Today, however, the Psychologist came to visit. I was too tired to talk, so she left. People keep coming and going, including my Consultant. He says that the duration of my stay raises issues of civil liberties, and that they couldn't keep me here forever. He wants me to live in some kind of "isolation in the community". He doesn't believe it's a good idea for me to go back home or to live with my partner. I can't believe our three-year relationship is going to take this turn. It's become impractical, in the face of infection control.

I don't know how I'm feeling now. I'm going to have to rebuild my life. This is hard when I don't know how or where I'm going to live.

The most important thing is quality of life, and I need to exercise freedom of choice. I can't help feeling that so much is being decided for me without my consultation. I don't want to be put on some council estate; forgotten, and struggling to survive on welfare.

A little later in the evening the Consultant came to my room. It seems I have misunderstood: I may be here for a very long time. It's still possible that I may not respond to the treatment: I may remain infectious. I may even die here.

Once again, I feel devastated. My hopes were so high. I thought I was seeing a light at the end of the tunnel. It was all my imagination. So, I've slipped back again into my world of hopelessness.

[Diary] Friday 25th August, 1995

My head is still swimming from the sedatives I took last night. I've filled the pee bottle and didn't know what to do with it. I'm so confused. There's a pain in my chest and it won't go away.

I can't go on like this. I've told the nurse that I'm going to refuse treatment, and have gone on hunger strike until something is done. They've got to give me a reason to live. I'm homeless, my three-year relationship is finished, I have nothing to go back to. Everything has been destroyed.

[Diary] Saturday 26th August, 1995

Perhaps I took a little too many sedatives last night- I feel groggy. I stood on the bed to open the roller blind and wobbled a bit; perhaps this sedation business isn't such a good idea after all.

Everyone's on holiday this weekend – it's a Bank Holiday. Looking out of the window, it seems the weather we've had over the last few weeks has gone on holiday as well. A typical, rainy British Bank Holiday weekend.

One of the nurses went to see how the work was going on my room. I may be able to move back in today, but as everyone knows, builders and deadlines don't always go hand in hand. I really hope I can move back. I haven't had a shower for three days.

Thankfully, she came back with good news. I can move back in today! We had a chat for a while, and I expressed the unfairness I felt at being here. I feel I've lost all sense of dignity. I used to think that the worst thing that could happen to anyone was to be locked up. Well, now it's happened to me, and it's hell.

Apparently, a few days ago, I'd frightened the nurses. I don't remember the incident. I'd asked one of them if I was already dead and said that I couldn't remember how I'd died. "It must have been quick, like a car crash." My mental state is deteriorating, an effect of being isolated.

I'm back in my old room. It has a phone now. It crackles a bit, not anyone's fault, just teething problems, I guess. The air extraction unit has added to the constant white noise there seems to be in the room. Along with the ticking of the bloody clock on the wall, it's quite noisy.

One of my visitors has brought in a personal stereo and some tapes. I'm listening to them now, and it's lifting my spirits. I want to survive – I want to live so much. I swing from one extreme to the other.

[Diary] Sunday 27th August, 1995

I sat around doing nothing today, just watching TV and trying not to think too much. My mind is my worst enemy sometimes. It causes me to say and do stupid things. Restraining tongue and pen is not always a bad idea. I was horrible to one of the nurses yesterday. I told her that I could kill her if I wanted to: then what would they do? LOCK ME UP? It had really frightened her, so I was glad to see her when she came in with a cup of tea for me. I reminded her of what I'd said and apologised. I don't know what gets into me sometimes! Anything that gives me a sense of control in a situation where it seems I have none seems like fair game right now.

I really don't know how to express the sadness I feel. Between the buildings outside I can see a small square of sky with a few tower blocks in the background. I know that out there the world still revolves, and people are getting on with their lives. I know that if I ever get out of here, I'm sure I will be grateful for those little things that we usually take for granted: my own bed, my own tea mug, my cat, if I can one day return to my life.

It doesn't matter what anyone says to me. Words mean nothing if you don't have your freedom. Oh, I don't know what I'm talking about. I don't even recognise my own confusion, perhaps even madness, anymore. I just don't recognise myself, period! I must rely on other people to tell me when I've lost it. But who could be that honest?

[Diary] Monday 28th August, 1995

I've never really liked Bank Holidays very much. That's probably my fault for not trying hard enough to do anything with them.

I had my traditional freezing cold shower this morning. I'm doing my best to try and keep fit. Yesterday, I even managed a few press-ups. I'm not going to push it today; I'll try and do some more tomorrow. I can feel the effect of them under my arms. Today, I'm going to pay attention to my legs. Perhaps some running on the spot or stretching exercises? Tomorrow, I might try some dreaded sit-ups, an exercise that I've never enjoyed doing because of the stomach ache it gives you. Then I'll go back to press-ups, afterwards, the legs, and back to the stomach, and so on.

Perhaps I've lost all sense of perspective. I seem to swing between the paranoia of being locked up in here forever to feelings of total euphoria. I sometimes feel like a worthless piece of shit, and that this episode in my life is going to have an unhappy ending. It's at times like this that I feel suicidal. That wouldn't solve anything, I know. I must try to think of ways to make myself feel better.

I must be constructive and make the best possible use of time. I have a friend in the Queen's Guard who's going to devise a fitness programme for me. He's going to bring in some weights for me. I've asked the nurses if I can use the exercise bike that I noticed on the ward. They don't see why not: it doesn't get used very much.

I'm also going to ask my doctor if I can have a sunbed. Hey, I can have a tan too! It could be that my skin may never feel the sun on it again. This would be the next best thing. Yeah, let's see how I can make the best of this time.

[Diary] Tuesday 29th August, 1995

Today is overcast. I love the sun. Through the bars at my window, I can see the cloudy sky and the old buildings of the hospital, with a newer one in the background. The nurse informed me it was a block of flats that was very popular for suicides because of its height. Way to go! I'm feeling a bit flat this morning. It may, however, be an interesting day; the hospital springs back into life after the Bank Holiday weekend, and the Consultant is coming around. In the meantime, I'm going to try to keep to my routine by having a cold shower, cleaning my teeth, getting dressed and doing my new fitness workout.

I've just weighed myself and I have put on 1kg! I'm now 61.1kg. When I was admitted, I was about 59kg. Very slim for even a skinny guy like me. I'd like to be back up to my normal weight of 68kg. That's what I was about a year ago. I've never been heavier than that anyway.

I had one of 'those' chats with a nurse. I went on about my fear of never getting out of the room. I pray to the God I hate and don't think exists that there'll be some progress soon.

[Diary] Wednesday 30th August, 1995

After I got up, I did 15 minutes on the exercise bike and I feel surprisingly good. Perhaps there's something in this exercise schtick after all? I like to try and shake off the 'cobwebs' left by the medication and sedatives they gave me last night.

I had a very unusual and moving discussion with one of the domestics who cleaned my room today. Her three-and-a-half-year-old son had been murdered. I found myself getting very emotional; it reminded me (temporarily) that I wasn't the only one having a very hard time. You lose sense of perspective when all you have is your imagination for company. I knew that underneath her orange mask she was smiling fondly at the memory of her child, sitting there on the edge of the bed with a duster in her hand. She shows no bitterness; she even believes it was an act of God. If it was, it fits in with my perception of Him, Her, It, Whatever. She says her life must go on.

I've used the exercise bike again; then 10 press-ups, and 10 of the dreaded sit-ups in the way my friend has shown me. I'm still waiting for the weights to arrive. I was half-asleep when the Consultant came in. He said it looked as though I was getting better and that, theoretically, I could leave if I could find somewhere suitable to live. I suppose by "suitable" he means in isolation. I would have to live under similar conditions to the ones I'm subjected to here. Same thing, a different place.

[Diary] Thursday 31st August, 1995

I woke up with what felt like a hangover this morning. But I've drunk nothing. I had my cold shower and once again forced myself to do some exercise.

A little later, the magnitude of the problems I'm facing began to dawn on me again. I was unable to return home or to mix with other people and perhaps would never be able to go out again. What's going to happen to me? I'm so frightened. Perhaps I shouldn't fight it; just accept that my life has been destroyed. If there is a future for me, it's likely to be very different. Today, I don't feel that I'm coping very well.

I have a slight pain in my chest that will hopefully pass. One of my visitors seems to know more about what's going on than I do.

Once again, I ritually close my orange blinds. I wonder if they'll throw them away when I leave? Maybe it'll all get burnt and I'll be in a bio-hazard body bag? The only time I seem to get any peace is when I'm asleep. This is so sad – I so used to enjoy life, when sleep was an inconvenient necessity that I endured, waiting for the next exciting day. Now, sleep is something I look forward to. It's a place where in my dreams I can go outside.

[Diary] Friday 1st September, 1995

I open my eyes and look at the clock. I've woken up very early again. It's about 4.30am. The sleeping pills only seem to cover me for about four hours these days. I thought about getting some more diazepam and just sleeping for a few more hours.

Before I got up, I pressed the red button for a cup of tea. The nurse who brought it in looked very tired from her night shift. She told me that things had really got moving since I'd been there. Doctors in general hadn't realised the potential problem that TB might present.

Fifteen minutes on the bike and a traditional cold shower. My stamina is increasing and soon I'll be able to use the weights.

LATER...

The day is turning into a bad one: I can feel the anger building in me. The doctor who I'd shouted at the other day came to see me. I apologised. Then, minutes later, another doctor came to see me. I questioned him about when I'd be able to go. He said that I might have to spend the rest of my life in this room. To say I lost it would be an understatement. I screamed at him, "If you're going to treat me like an animal, then I shall behave like one!" With that, I threw a jug of water at him. This narrowly missed him and shattered on the radiator opposite. He left the room saying he would come back when I had calmed down.

FUCK YOU, BUDDY!

[Diary] Saturday 2ⁿᵈ, September, 1995

The sedation has worn off. I can't sleep, and they won't give me more. There's no point in wishing for the day when I'll be free again. They say I must stay here because it's in the wider interests of public health. I don't know where I'm at; my profound determination to live turns into suicidal depression, and the swing can happen in seconds.

[Diary] Monday 11ᵗʰ September, 1995

The usual pattern of me waking up about 4am, having had a night sweat, and with a soaked pair of pyjamas and sheets has become familiar. Dazed, I generally sit there in my armchair while the nurses change my sheets.

I've had my workout. I've got my new weights now, and I feel I'm getting stronger. A whole load of letters have arrived for me.

[Letter] Monday 11ᵗʰ September, 1995

Dear Paul,

By now you have probably been deluged with mail in response to the article in last week's edition of THUD. *I hope that you've got time to read another!*

By now you will have realized that there was

one thing wrong about what was written. You may be forced to be alone physically, but you are not alone in spirit. There are a lot of people thinking about you, including me. I can only vaguely appreciate what you must be going through and would not pretend to think otherwise. I have spent periods of time alone, out of choice, and am aware that it can sometimes be a depressing experience.

I can't really understand why you are not allowed visitors or been given better facilities; I appreciate that the MDR-TB might be a risk for certain people, but this should not stop them from seeing you, if they really want to. It should not stop the hospital authorities from treating you with the respect that we all deserve, regardless of our medical status or physical condition. If you are short of visitors, and would be happy to welcome another, not as someone just to talk to, but as a friend, then I would be very happy to see you. I am HIV-negative, in excellent health, and not suffering from any other ailments that I am aware of. My last boyfriend told me that he was a Hepatitis B carrier as soon as we met and insisted that I get vaccinated against the virus. Anyway, I've had a number of shots and still come back Hep B negative. I've got the final six-

month shot due in early October. I don't know if this would bar me from visiting you, but as far as I'm concerned, I'm quite happy taking the risk.

I don't know if you would even want any more visitors, so, again, I'd be pleased to correspond with you, if you have had the time and energy to spare (and inclination!). By the way I am not a handwriting snob, but if you saw mine you really would be horrified and appalled. As I have access to a PC with decent WP facilities, I figure I might as well take advantage of them. I can also get more on the page this way.

I do hope you are in good spirits, or at least as good as possible, in spite of this letter. I have never been so moved as to put pen to paper, so to speak, so this is the first for me, and I apologize if it has come out somewhat clumsily and stilted, I am not so hot on contrived spontaneity. At least it should be legible.

Take care, and hope to speak to you sometime.

All the best,

F.T., London SW8

[Letter] Monday 11th September, 1995

Dear Paul,

I recently read an article about you.

I'm 23 and scared to death that I may be HIV-positive. I'm just too frightened to get tested and facing the outcome. I worry about this all of the time (I just felt like sharing this with you). After reading about you and your circumstances I had to write and send a small chocolate-filled token – so you know that others are thinking about you even if they don't know you... wow!

I am sending some information about you and the article to the US. So you may start getting post from worldwide.

You are definitely in my Roman Catholic prayers and thoughts.

C.P., London N22

[Letter] Tuesday 12th September, 1995

Dear Paul,

I have read about your incredibly difficult situation with the drug-resistant TB infection, and currently having to live in isolation. I'm sorry that things are not good at the moment as regards your healthcare arrangements. I do hope that the health authority can make some sort of better arrangements for you soon.

After reading about your story, I thought I would write to you and offer my meagre support on paper.

I will tell you something about myself briefly to introduce myself. My name is Brendan; I'm 30 years old (gay, of course) and work for local government as a social worker with children and families. I too, like yourself, love chocolate, and I am a definite chocoholic who desperately needs rehabilitation from this dreadful addiction.

If you love chocolate so much I will try to leave some chocolate for you on the ward if they will allow me (maybe you will write and tell me what bars you like?). I hope that you are provided with lots of chocolate bars by many of those generous gay boys (and gals) out there. You are probably in the hearts and prayers of many of us out here, and I hope we can do something to help change your situation.

Paul, please try and have faith in the love of your gay and lesbian community. (I hope you do, so I'm sorry if that sounds patronizing; it's not my intention.) I really believe that it can sustain you during this time of trial. I can never imagine quite *what being in isolation feels like for you, but I do hope I can try to have some understanding and that will enable me to try and do something practical / political, to help you. I will try to investigate what I can do to support yourself and other positive people in your situation, in whatever way I can – I hope you don't mind (if you do, let me know).*

Well, Paul, I won't say too much. I will continue to write to you (unless I hear from you and you tell me to bugger off).

Take care, God bless and protect you,

From Brendan M., London, SE1

P.S.   I enclose an SAE in case you are short of stamps.

[Letter] Tuesday 12th September, 1995

Dear Paul,

I have never felt compelled to write to someone after reading their story, but yours touched me like no other. I cannot pretend, even to imagine what you must be going through. Hopefully, as a result of the article in 'Thud', loads of people will have written to you and you will know that people you have never met do care and are thinking of you. It's a shame we can't visit you – or can we?

I will keep this letter short as no doubt the deluge of mail will abate somewhat and to write to you when you will have time to read it! If there are any books or magazines or whatever that you want, let me know and I will see what I can do.

Best Wishes,

P.H., London N21

P.S. My contribution to the first EEC chocolate mountain – what do you really like? I imagine in a few weeks all the nurses will have put on half a stone – you will be popular!

[Diary] Friday 15th September, 1995

For the last four days I've been in tortured limbo. A 'no-man's land'. The Living Dead. I haven't worked out, written, read or done anything else. I've turned away visitors, and I seem to have just withdrawn into myself. I don't know what happened. Perhaps I just blew a fuse of sorts? I don't think I've ever been that depressed before. Today, I feel a bit more normal. Whatever normal is! There are two men in my room; they arrived just after I woke up and have come to have another stab at fixing the shower.

The Consultant came in next. I wasn't expecting to see him so early. It was about 8.30am. He's flying off to the States today to find out more about this disease and wants to tie up any loose ends before he goes.

I often worry about the potential for infecting other people. I don't know whether I could live with this if it happened. I'm looking forward to the Consultant coming back from the US. He may have some good news for me? I must try to trust him; at times, his actions seem draconian, but they're well-intended. Faith, I suppose – a type of thinking I find hard to sustain.

[Letter] Friday 15th September, 1995

Dear Paul,

I hope that you received the chocolates and the Gay Times.

They tried to do the same thing to me as they have done to you, but I told them I am going home and I'm glad that I did as I am feeling a lot better, and I knew I would have just gone down-hill, as having people around who care about you is a bonus.

I will be going to the hospital on Tuesday, so I will bring in some more chocolates and sweets.

Well, keep fighting and don't let them think they

are winning.

Take care.

Yours,

T.G., London E15

[Diary] Sunday 17th September, 1995

Would you believe it! There has been an outbreak of scabies on the ward. Most of the nurses looking after me have it and have passed it on to other patients. On close inspection, it seems I have it too. So much for isolation! I've been itching quite a bit, come to think of it. I feel so dirty already, what with the TB and HIV. I am filth.

Once again, I'm finding it difficult to cope. I want to throw something through the window or make a dash for the door. How can they punish me? What more can they do? However, doing this now may jeopardise any chances I have of being discharged. If I'm co-operative now they may be more inclined to let me go sometime in the future?

[Diary] Monday 18th September, 1995

I've become so selfish being here; I've been unable to think about anything else except my predicament. I have a friend who's been ill for quite a long time with a brain tumour. They tried to operate, but only managed to remove 80% of it. His chances of survival are not good, apparently. He's on a lot of medication that has made his face swell up. I'm told by my friends that it's hard to recognise him now.

I love my friend James dearly. I wish I could see him. I just don't know why this has happened to him. He isn't HIV-positive, like me. He's a 25-year-old man, just like me, with everything going for him. It's so unfair. Perhaps I deserve this disease? He doesn't deserve his.

I dowsed myself in the lotion I'd been given to kill the scabies. It stinks. Just another ritual I've added to my daily routine. I have to say, it doesn't smell very nice at all. I've had to cover myself from head to foot. All my clothes have been taken away to be washed, and my sheets have been changed. Scabies – just another one of the lovely social diseases that I seem to be making a habit of collecting. In the meantime, I'm walking about holding up some very large pyjamas; otherwise, they just fall off me, as I have no clothes.

My thoughts are racing. I'm in between two worlds. Neither dead nor alive.

[Letter] Monday 18th September, 1995

Dear Paul,

It's been a little while since I last heard from you, and I'm hoping it's because you've been busy communicating with lots of other people, and not because you've been ill or too depressed to write.

I know that it's very hard on you; you've got people around you who are unwell, and may not last as long as you, there are numerous times when you yourself are physically ill or in pain, and that's hard too, but you must never give up on yourself. Even if you have, there are lots of other people out there who haven't given up on you (like me!).

Let me tell you a little about what's been happening to me. Since I last wrote, work got very busy, and left me running around like the proverbial blue-arsed fly. I've no love life at the moment (much to my chagrin; more on that in due course), so I tend to focus on work rather than play. As you can imagine, too much running around is not good for you, and sure enough I caught a flu bug that's been going around. This one seems to be particularly virulent; I was laid low for well over a week, and could hardly get out of bed (I know it's nothing compared to what you've had to experience, but it felt pretty serious to me!). A good friend of mine went to the chemist and stocked up on a little pharmacy for me: cough mixtures, cold powders, flu capsules, throat lozenges, multi-vitamins, and lots of orange juice and canned soups. I couldn't eat properly for the first week and managed to lose 5lbs (if your unlucky enough to see me in person, or a photo, you'll realize that I can't afford to lose any more weight), which is slowly coming back.

Needless to say, my friends all told me it's my own fault for working too hard, and that I need a good man to keep an eye on me! Ha!

So, with a little encouragement, and confidence-building from friends, I've sent off a few letters to some of the Personal columns in the gay press. I hasten to add that I'm going for the 1-2-1 relationship. I'm not into one-night stands, and all the shallow things that the scene seems to bring out in some people.

My last boyfriend was someone I met under quite romantic circumstances through friends of mine. Just over Easter, a couple whom I've been good friends with for a number of years invited me over for a dinner party the following Sunday. When I arrived, there were just two other guests, Jacqui, straight but very gay-friendly, and Andrew.

At dinner, Andrew and I were seated opposite one another, and the conversation seemed to be manipulated so that we spoke together a great deal, and it was also revealed that we were both single. Needless to say, we exchanged a lot of glances over dinner, and when the party broke up, and we all went our separate ways, Andrew and I exchanged telephone numbers, and ended up in contact mid-morning the following day (which, thankfully, was a Bank Holiday). Anyway, Andrew came over to my flat and we talked and talked and talked for hours (at least six or seven), and after a while, he asked me if I would "go out" with him. My goodness, how corny and romantic! I was so flattered and honest.

It sounds like the perfect meeting, and that we ought to live happily ever after, but as we both know, life isn't always like that, and as time went on we realized that we wanted different things from our relationship and that we were unable to reconcile certain fundamental differences. After three and a half months we finally split, somewhat acrimoniously as well. After a period of non-communication, we have finally become friends (albeit cautious on my side!) and speak on the phone once every two or three weeks. I have even put some business his way, so I guess I have learnt not to allow myself to become emotionally prejudiced.

It was my first proper relationship for nearly three years (the previous one lasted for nearly three years, but that is another story for another time).

Now I'm looking again, but not too hard, and I'm not expecting anything wonderful to happen straight away. My beloved Wicked Stepmother told me recently that the right guy will come along, not necessarily sooner rather than later, and maybe not in the shape or form or circumstances that I would expect, but that when it happens I'll definitely know about it!

Enough from me for now, it's over to you. Even if you don't feel like writing anything about yourself, just a short note, to let me know that this letter has vaguely cheered and amused and not left you bored? Let me know that you're doing OK; if you are not, then let me know what's been affecting you, and what I can do to help.

Anyway, do take care, and don't be unhappy; I'm thinking of you and rooting for you.

F.T., London SW8

[Diary] Tuesday 19th September, 1995

Not good today. Should I stop taking the medication? More questions for which I don't have the answers. I apply a funny sort of logic; If I am to spend the rest of my life in this room, then I think I'd rather die. Of course, suicide is an option and crosses my mind frequently: I often think about how I might go about it. The thing that really holds me back is cowardice. I just can't do it.

After all these dark thoughts, my mind seems to dwell on the things I would miss. Then I yearn for them and become excited once more about being released. Suddenly, I feel quite hopeful again. I swing wildly from the dreams of a new life to the nightmare of the old one.

However, I feel like fighting most of the time. If only out of curiosity to see what will happen.

[Diary] Wednesday 20th September, 1995

My sunbed arrived today!

[Diary] Thursday 21st September, 1995

I woke up early and had my usual cup of tea and cigarettes, thinking about the day ahead. My hair's getting rather long and needs cutting. However, the hospital hairdresser can only do a 'blue rinse and set' by all accounts, and I don't think it'll suit me!

I opened the blinds when I was cleaning my teeth, and just stood there wide-eyed. There were two huge magpies sitting on the roof opposite. I could see right into their eyes. I felt so excited at seeing them that I spat out the toothpaste and rushed over to the nurses call button. I wanted at least one of them to see them. These things have become so important to me: the first day in isolation seems an eternity away.

I waited for the nurse to come, hoping that they wouldn't fly away in the meantime. One of them moved out of view as she came through the door. "Look," I said, pointing through the window. She was startled to say least: "Don't show me that – I don't want to see one of them!" I was confused; she told me that to see one of these birds on its own was said to be unlucky and could bring great sorrow. Two, on the other hand, was a good omen. I had seen two. It is probably foolish to put faith in such things, but it certainly made me feel better.

Two of the doctors came to see me. Apparently, my 'liver function tests' are abnormal. Not surprising, really, considering the amount of medication that I'm taking. One of the doctors examined my stomach. In his opinion, there was nothing going on that was too serious. However, they decided to carry out a scan of my abdomen.

Come to think of it, I'd had some stomach pains over the last few weeks. I put this down to my new fitness routine and had blamed the dreaded sit-ups. The doctors also told me that they weren't sure if I was getting better. Strange, because I feel okay. They say I should be smear-negative by now, but according to the recent samples this is not the case. If things haven't changed by next Monday, they're going to try a new drug.

I really don't want any more drugs. The doctor's going to consult another hospital about the new drug to see how effective it is. They haven't used it before here.

I've asked my friend to bring in my Polaroid camera. I'm going to make a montage of my room. Although it's small, there could be a lot of good photos. A small art project, perhaps? At least it's something to do. One of the things I really hate is asking people for help when they may reply in the negative. I don't like being dependent on others, and I don't like the thought of them saying "no".

Later in the day, my friend came to see me with the camera. I experimented with a few pictures of the bars at my window and other things that would remain evocative of my 'residence'. The world as I knew it.

[Diary] Friday 22nd September, 1995

Today has been dull and uneventful, except that I've been told there will be a case conference about me next Friday. I am not invited. I feel angry that I'm not able to be involved with the decisions which are being made about my life. Complaining about my loss of human rights seems to make no difference. Let them decide whatever, I'm just going to try and get on with what I need to do to stay alive.

Another week gone has gone by. I've tried to keep busy. The weekend is here, that silent time when the hospital seems to sleep, and those who work here go home to their own lives after interfering with everybody else's.

[Diary] Saturday 23rd September, 1995

I've decided to try and have a "Be Nice to Paul day". Sunbeds, fitness and rest. My hair is pissing me off! It hasn't been this long for ages, and I'm apprehensive about the blue-rinse brigade. I've asked a friend to buy some hair clippers and I'm going to chop it all off.

Well, I've done it. Now I have no hair at all! (I got a bit carried away!)

[Letter] Saturday 23rd September, 1995

Dear Paul,

I hope you will not mind me writing to you, but what with everything in the press recently I couldn't just ignore it and not make some contact with you. It goes without saying that I am extremely upset and angry to hear about what has happened to you, and the articles I have read have really got to me and I'm sure must have touched the hearts of all that read it. It's very difficult to know what to say to you at this stage other than my thoughts are with you and I would be very happy to hear from you should you wish to write back. I'll therefore keep this letter very brief until I've heard from you.

In the meantime, don't give up, Paul. Everyone I have spoken to (friends and family) have been shocked and dismayed to hear of your predicament and I'm sure there will be growing pressure to improve your circumstances. Please write back soon and I'll promise to reply with a longer letter once I have heard from you.

Best wishes,

Terry M., London N15

[Letter] Saturday 23rd September, 1995

Dear Paul,

Many thanks for your letter. I hope you enjoyed the chocolates I left for you on the ward?

Well, I will be writing to my MP about how outrageous your current care deal is, and I will be writing to a MEP. I am encouraging my friends to do the same. I did not want to express too much outrage in my initial letter to you, however, after your reply, I now feel okay about being frank. Quite honestly, I think it is disgraceful that the medical profession hasn't seen further than providing an isolation room to meet your needs. I think what you said about the UK being unable to deal with MDR-TB is very worrying! Ethics need to accompany medical care for anyone, and it seems that as far as this infection is concerned, ethics don't come into it. I will try to do something to address this injustice and *encourage others to do the same. I'm pleased that what I wrote about the support of the lesbian and gay community helped you. I think that in our community there are many of us who are gifted and loving people, and we are a tower of strength to each other. You come across as being a vibrant, strong and loving individual who has stood up to a great deal of difficulty and pain and who still bares much. I don't know if I would have been able to cope so well if I had to go through some of the trials you have endured.*

I'll come to a close for now. Take care of yourself and please do feel supported. I will write again soon.

God Bless.

B., London, SE1

[Letter] Wednesday 27th September, 1995

Dear Paul,

Like many people I had heard about a TB outbreak in a West London hospital, but nothing of the people involved.

I read about you in Positive Nation *and thought about writing to you immediately, however, on giving it more thought, I could think of little to say, in fear of saying the wrong thing or appearing naïve.*

This is how I first felt when I first became a volunteer at the Hillingdon AIDS Response Trust. Probably because I am a straight female, and also because I felt there was little I could actually do to help. I have learnt since then that an open mind, honesty and the ability to listen and support enables me to help.

I wouldn't dream of saying that I understand what it is to live with HIV/AIDS, but through the friendships I have made through HART, I know something of the emotions associated with it.

Your situation is obviously different to the people I know with HIV/AIDS because of your isolated environment; although you are alone, people have read of your situation, people are aware of how you are living and people care.

Lots of love,

S.M., Middlesex, UB7

[Diary] Thursday 28th September, 1995

I hate this room. My window is so dirty; I can barely see the dismal view of the brick wall outside. In the distance nothing moves on the motorway. There is nothing. I must prop the door of the bathroom open with the handle of a mop. The drain of the shower stinks, and I have no option but to breath in the stench. I will probably catch something else at this rate. MDR-TB, scabies – I hate to think what other possibilities lurk in here!

[Letter] Thursday 28th September, 1995

Dear Paul,

Do you remember me? I'm Terry's Mum. You spent Christmas 1988 with us and fed Ben his dinner. He was 9 months old then and his is now 7½.

We were all shocked when Terry phoned to convey the news of your illness. We all spoke of the times you spent here with Terry and the photos you took in Amsterdam.

We have obviously read various items in the press regarding you and your condition, and it is unbelievable in this day and age that this was allowed to happen.

Ben now has a brother, Joe, who will be five in two weeks' time. Do you remember Terry's brother Alan and his wife Janice? They have two children now. Daniel is 4 and Hannah is 2½. Terry's youngest brother, Philip, has bought a house in

Milton Keynes, but he isn't married yet. I am still working at the elderly people's home, and I am now the manager. I have been there 25 years now.

I understand you are on the television in the early hours of Saturday morning, so I will be recording it. We have got you on video giving Ben his bottle of milk. Do you remember?

I do hope you don't mind me writing to you Paul? Over the last few years Terry's Dad and myself understand so much more about the gay community, much more than we ever did – all thanks to Terry, who has spent many an hour talking to us.

Do write back if you want. I wish you all the luck, and remember there are a lot of people thinking of you.

Regards,

Sylvia and Bill M.

[Diary] Friday 29th September, 1995

There's going to be another case conference about me on the ward today. As I shan't be present (again), I have issued a statement to be read by someone else on my behalf. This is to remind them that it's my life they're making decisions about. I can't help feeling that the mistakes that were made at the beginning of the HIV epidemic are about to be made again. Everyone seems so frightened by the threat I apparently pose to others.

The conference started at around 2pm. I really don't know what was said. As far as I can ascertain, it amounted to nothing more than the people involved getting better acquainted. No real decisions were made. It has taken so long to get them around a table together, and yet the most important person, my Consultant, wasn't even there. He is still in the States. Once again it seems I shall have to wait.

The minutes have turned to hours, and I can hear the ticking of the clock on the wall. The time between each second seems to be getting longer. I sometimes just lie here, my hopes fading, trying desperately to find the strength to go on. I've tried doing everything I can. It is possible I'm going to lose this battle.

[Letter] Friday 29ᵗʰ September, 1995

Dear Paul,

I hope you don't mind me writing to you. I have just been listening to your story on The James Whale Show, *and what a story! It's unbelievable in this day* and age that this can be allowed to happen. It left me shocked and angry. Through no fault of your own, you are in prison, but even real prisoners get a reprieve. My prison is my body. I have a degenerative spinal disease which over the years has crushed my wild child spirit and forced it into submission. Like you, I have the outward appearance of a normal person who is fit and well. Like you, I have a small gym in my room which not only guards against wasting muscles but perpetuates a feeling of wellbeing and health. Like you, my youth has been stolen from me. People tell me how brave I am, but I don't feel brave, just angry. I don't know about you, but I find this situation tends to make one less idealistic and more realistic about human nature and life. I'm sure that, like me, you are under no illusions about the many failings of our fellow man.

I don't mean to sound bitter. To the outside world I appear happy and even-tempered, even sweet. I write my thoughts and feelings in this letter only by way of an explanation as to why I feel some sort of understanding of what you might be going through, albeit in a very small way, compared to your situation.

I have no political power, nor money, so I can't help you in any material way. Even so, I very much hope you will write back to me and tell me a little about yourself. To be honest, I'm not even sure what made me write to you, I just felt that I had to write.

I look forward to hearing from you.

Cindy F., Manchester

[Letter] Friday 29th September, 1995

Dear Paul,

It feels rather strange writing this letter – for two reasons. Firstly, I don't know if this letter will even reach you, and secondly, to be frank, I am completely clueless as to what to say!

I heard your story on The James Whale Show *and felt moved to send you a note (via the programme – I just hope they forward it!) in the hope that for at least a few seconds I can relieve you from the unimaginable emotions that you must be going through.*

Obviously, I know nothing at all of your circumstances and, to be honest, I'm having great difficulty trying to get my head around what you are experiencing – being 27 myself, I simply cannot begin to imagine what it must be like for you.

What impressed me about you on the programme was the concern that you conveyed about the other people who are predicted of contracting TB over the coming years, and your apparent lack of bitterness towards the situation you yourself are in. You are obviously someone who has an incredibly strong character – it really was incredibly humbling to hear your story.

There are obviously thousands of horror stories that we are bombarded with on a day-by-day basis, but I can honestly say that yours has definitely moved me more than any other. I can't exactly say why – perhaps it's the unfairness of it. I think it is probably because I feel completely inadequate and totally unable to help or even grasp what it must be like for you.

You know – I started this letter with every intention of being "deep" and so far, I have completely failed!!

Well, if we were face-to-face I suppose I'd tell you a bit about myself (and find out about you, which obviously isn't possible!) so at the risk of boring you witless, I'll introduce myself. Hi, I'm Pete. Like I said, I'm 27 – I'm engaged to Mandy and we have a seven-year-old daughter, Danielle. I have my own business and Mandy works in a bank. I enjoy reading, listening to music (everything from Vivaldi to Metallica – a bit strange, I know!) and sport, watching rather than participating. So that's me!

Anyway, Paul – I'll sign off now – I am not that practiced at letter writing. I sincerely wish you all the very best and hope that the people responsible for your current position can get you out of it.

Words just don't seem enough somehow. I wish I could express how I feel, but I can't. Suffice to say I don't see me sleeping tonight. Your story has totally done my head in, for want of a better phrase. Stay positive, never give up, stay strong for yourself.

I will probably never know whether this letter reaches you. I truly hope that it does and that in some miniscule way it helps you to know that a complete stranger is thinking of you.

My Best wishes,

Pete M., Great Yarmouth

[Letter] Friday 29th September, 1995

Dear Paul,

Really pleased to hear that my letter came as a pleasant surprise and that many others have taken the time to write to you. Yes, you're right, there are lots of selfish bastards in this world (I've met most of them!), but there are also a surprising number of genuine people who do care about others and not just themselves. I am also very glad to hear that you are not suffering too much physically although the mental strain caused by your isolation etc. must be almost unbearable at times.

Well, now I have an opportunity to bore you with a brief resume of my life over the past few years. I'm not going to dwell too much on the four and a half years I spent with Steve (the guy I went out with after you), as my life was extremely complicated during most of that time by his perpetual alcoholism. I am not bitter or resentful about my time with Steve; it goes without saying that I learnt a great deal about life and people during that time (albeit, the hard way) which I now believe has benefited me since. I still sympathise with his situation which I now understand will be with him for the rest of his life, but I am glad not to be part of it anymore. Partly because of Steve's problem and partly due to my own stupidity I ended up in several thousand pounds worth of debt which, thankfully, now is greatly reduced. My relationship with Steve ended by him simply 'disappearing' one day without a word (having allegedly committed a fairly minor crime) and I was left to pick up the pieces. I didn't hear from him again for about three months so, as you can imagine, this was a very difficult time for me.

In January 1994, my 'new life' began by meeting a very special guy who was to become my boyfriend, Darren. You may remember meeting him briefly outside Compton's bar that last time I saw you. We have now been together for 19 months and moved into a flat together in June 1994. It's a Victorian house converted into two flats and we live on the first floor. We have three bedrooms, and the garden at the back of the house is divided into two with steps leading down from our kitchen. It's not a bad area to live in, although there has recently been a problem with prostitution so most evenings the street corners are attended by various prossies and their pimps (but no rent-boys, unfortunately!). I still own a house in Stevenage which I bitterly regret buying and is rented out as I am unable to sell it and have about ten thousand pounds worth of negative equity on it.

Darren (or 'Daz') is, like you, 24, and to put it simply we are very much in love with each other.

Daz works as a foreign exchange cashier for American Express (and formerly, Thomas Cook) which means we have had several excellent cheap holidays together. He also gets a few "educational tours" which only travel industry staff can travel on, so last year he went to Barbados and next week he is on a whistle-stop tour to Los Angeles, Las Vegas, the Grand Canyon etc. (Bastards!!). Still "while the cat's away...", I shall be hopefully having some fun on my own! I can't really complain, though, in all the time I spent with Steve we only managed one holiday; since being with Daz we have been to Turkey, Morocco, France, Germany, Switzerland, Luxembourg and Copenhagen. Next year we are hoping to visit Thailand.

I met Daz at Turnmills and when we go clubbing we enjoy Trade more than anywhere else. Other than going to Trade about once a month we rarely visit other clubs, although we still go to Soho for a drink occasionally. I really fell for him from day one, and pestered the life out of him to go out with me and eventually he gave in. Of course, he soon realised what a 'catch' I was and now he loves me almost as much as I love him. We are both very open and honest with each other and managed to stay monogamous and faithful for the first year although we now have an 'open relationship' within certain rules, which we review from time to time. This has caused its problems in trying to get the balance right, but we both agreed from day one that we would both need a certain amount of freedom at some later stage and we have therefore been adjusting to this over the past few months.

I also have a chocolate-brown Labrador dog named Emma whom I have had since a puppy and who will be six years old in November (this made our first flat hunting a little more difficult last year as we had to have a place with a garden). She is a complete lunatic and a big softy, but generally well-behaved and loving. She also provides a certain amount of security for the flat and ourselves which makes up for being 'tied down' to a certain extent by having a dog. Fortunately, we have a couple of friends who are only too willing to look after her when we go on holidays, during which she also has a good time as they thoroughly spoil her and she gets fatter every time we leave her. So that's my little family which I hope one day you will be well enough to come and meet.

As for my 'extended family', they are all well

and still living in Stevenage with the exception of my younger brother, Phil, who now lives in Milton Keynes and is the only one of my three brothers still unmarried, although I think most of our suspicions regarding his sexuality have now been ruled out! If he is gay he must be firmly in the closet or completely wasting his life. My mum and dad actually plucked up the courage to ask him outright a couple of years ago, which I think quite shocked him. I now have three nephews and one niece; you may recall my eldest nephew, Ben, from the Christmas you spent with me at Stevenage. He is now seven (I think?), and growing up to be a very cute boy as is his very cheeky younger brother Joe.

My dad finally retired from work this year at the age of 66 and despite his misgivings to start with seems to have settled quite happily into his new life with lots of time on his hands. He is not the kind of person to sit around doing nothing, though, so he keeps himself very busy around the house and garden and also does some community work. My mum is now manager of the old peoples' home where she first started working part-time as a care assistant over 25 years ago and enjoys her work very much. For some time, she was deputy manager *under another woman who she became good friends with and who is a lesbian, so I think she has learnt even more about homosexuality and our lifestyles from her. My dad, surprisingly, has also become very relaxed about my sexuality and much more open to discussion. He avidly watches any gay TV programme and reads the gay newspapers I take home for him occasionally.*

I'm still working for the same lousy company, doing pretty much the same job except that these days I mostly service the retail sector, so I get to fix tills as well as computers (impressive, huh?!). It's not exactly awe inspiring and I have no career objectives at all, but it pays very well for what I do and at least I can completely 'switch off' from work each day. I am based at home and my calls are almost exclusively within the M25. I rarely go into the office and most days I get home for lunch, which is useful as Emma doesn't then get left alone all day. I also get the occasional quiet day at home (like today) when there might only be one or two calls, or even none at all. When they eventually make me redundant, which could be tomorrow, next month, or next year, I'll start thinking about what I really want to do.

So, how about you, Paul? What's been happening in your life apart from the obvious? Not all bad, I hope. It sounds like things were working out for you before this recent turn of events.

I look forward to hearing from you again in due course and if there is anything more I can do for you, please let me know. I hope that your recovery continues and that you will soon be out of there.

Love and Best wishes,

Terry M.

[Letter] Saturday 30ᵗʰ September, 1995

Dear Paul,

I cannot find words to express my sorrow for your predicament. Some believe that our futures are mapped out. Destiny, if you like, but some don't.

I feel that there is a destiny for every person. I cannot knowledgably comment on your destiny; however, I have a little story about me and what is my destiny.   Here goes!

Aged 16 I was extremely introvert, but I got involved with drugs. Firstly cannabis for a couple of years, then the prescription drug temazepam and speed. I was then prescribed methadone (why methadone? I don't know why, because it is a cannabis substitute). Anyway, I came off the methadone in September 1990 (when my daughter was born). After coming off drugs I thought that I was chemically invincible (in other words I had taken just about everything and was still alright), but after roughly about 6 months I started taking speed again and after a couple more months (after taking a lot of speed again daily) instead of having a ball when I was out clubbing I was 100% paranoid and insecure. I thought it would go, but it didn't. For a couple of years, which sometimes felt like a lifetime, the paranoia continued (long after I had stopped taking speed). I went to Manchester for a year, no positive lifestyle – mainly alcohol, and I then came back to the Rhondda.

I started Kyokushin Karate as just about a down and out, but I persevered, sweated just about blood, and have dropped all of the drugs and have made myself both mentally and physically much stronger. Two weeks ago, I won the Welsh Karate Championships. I think my destiny includes Kyokushin Karate, whatever else. I would be very honored if you would take the time to write back to me.

M.W., Pontypridd

[Letter] Sunday 1st October, 1995

Dear Paul,

I am writing on behalf of my Mum. She has been suffering from MDR-TB for two years. She is in the City Hospital in Nottingham on an isolation ward.

My Mum couldn't really say much about what you said, but told me that your hospital room has bars on the windows and that you are not allowed out. We were beginning to think we were the only ones in the country with the disease, but obviously now we know there are more.

It would be a great help to Mum if you would write to her (I think she is writing to you herself, but it takes time for her to do anything). She has had a lung removed to try to help recovery and cure her of the disease and would really like to hear from you as extra support and hope.

Family members also suffer mentally because of our loved one's suffering, so if any of your family would like to write to me, I would be pleased to write back. We could form a support group of our own. It must help knowing there's someone else who knows exactly how you feel and understands what the families are going through.

She is fighting hard to beat this, and I hope you

feel that there is hope too.

We hope to hear from you very soon. My best wishes to you and your family.

V.S., Nottingham

[Diary] Monday 2nd October, 1995

Today could be an important day. My Consultant is back from his fact-finding mission to the States. Let's hope he has some new ideas. This last weekend really dragged. I'm much better physically since the Consultant last saw me. My weight has increased by 5kg. A very good sign. The fitness routine seems to have worked as well. I now have a 28-inch waist, and the belly that was there seems to have moved to my chest! The tan is coming on nicely. In fact, I can't remember the last time I looked this good. It remains to be seen what this week's sputum samples will show. I hope that the Consultant comes to see me soon. I feel calm, and for the first time in months I feel confident that I am winning this battle.

The Consultant came to see me about 5.45pm this evening. He said things which buoyed me up even further. It seems the trip to the States may have paid off after all. In the first instance, he says I look better than I did before he went away. More importantly, he seems to have made up his mind about the criteria for my release. If I achieve three negative sputum smear tests in the next three weeks I can go. He is going to sort out some accommodation that is suitable for me. It looks like I may be out of here soon. The last thing he told me was amazing: his trip to the US has changed things. So long as I comply with Direct Observed Therapy, attend the clinic at least once a month and remain sputum-negative, I will be able to lead a relatively normal life. The only thing I really mustn't do is spend time with immuno-compromised people.

I'm frightened. I've become used to living in isolation, and soon I am to be set free. It seems like quite a challenge, and the thought of an open space is very daunting.

[Letter] Monday 2ⁿᵈ October, 1995

Dear Paul,

I heard you talking on The James Whale Show *the other night and was completely gob-smacked that things like this can happen to people. I was fucking angry, and it isn't even happening to me. I dread to think how you feel. Anyway, you think you have got it bad. I've had to tape a Dolly Parton LP for my parents – now, that is torture!*

Well, I'm a student (yes, sponging off the state),
but I spend most of my time in the pub. I am only at
college, but hopefully I will get to university
eventually. I live in Birmingham (which is a really
sad place). I am finding this quite difficult because I
feel badly about telling you what I'm doing when
you don't have the same luxury. I'm not sure
whether this is what you really want to hear? But
anyway, I will plod on. I'm in a lot of pain now
because I kicked the bed really hard and it feels like I
have broken my toes. I can't even get my boots on
because I am in agony. So no going to the pub for
me today.

I'm a big film buff and I love music too. I want
to go and see Apollo 13. *My favorite films are* J.F.K,
Kalifornia, A Few Good Men, Dead Poet's Society,
Basic Instinct, Gone with the Wind – *and the list is*
endless. I like all kinds of music including Nirvana,
Pearl Jam, The Cranberries and some dance music.
What about you?

I'm 24, although you can probably tell that from
my appalling handwriting. I am also a girl. My
name is Julie. Not only that, but I am a gay girl. I
haven't got a girlfriend because I had my heart

broken about 6 months ago and I am not best pleased about it. So, women can go jump as far as I am concerned. Yes, I am all bitter and twisted! I HATE WOMEN!!

It must be hard for you to maintain any kind of relationship with anyone in the situation that you are in. Have you got a partner? What about family? Do you have any other support? Do you think the doctors are going to be able to cure you?

Anyhow, I assume that you are allowed to write letters. I hope I haven't bored you too much. If I have, just write back and tell me to piss off. I can take the rejection. I might kill myself – but that is not your concern. Ha!

Anyway, I hope that you are okay, and I hope to hear from you soon.

Love,

Julie, Birmingham

[Diary] Tuesday 3rd October, 1995

The weather is dismal – it's raining heavily. I completely missed the summer; I feel so much better when the sun shines. All I have in here is the constant flicker of an overhead fluorescent light. I feel a little depressed; this seems quite usual considering the time (about 5pm). I think this is because most of the people who help me have gone home and have probably forgotten about me – I'm just another part of their work.

[Diary] Friday 6th October, 1995

Something has got to give. I'm trying to find the strength from somewhere, but I feel I'm scraping the bottom of the barrel. I pace the floor like a caged animal in a zoo. The drains smell particularly bad today. The doctors and nurses come and go. All they ever give me is tea and pills. I'm sick of being a disease. I want to be a human being again.

[Diary] Saturday 7th October, 1995

I woke up and went through the ritual of getting dressed. I opened the blinds; the sun was shining for a change. I would really like to be out there. Instead I sit here resisting the temptation to watch kids' TV. There is absolutely nothing to do. I've listened to my CDs a hundred times or more.

[Diary] Monday 9th October, 1995

I woke up at about 8am and got showered and dressed. I threw a paper towel in the rubbish bin, which, as per usual, was overflowing after the weekend. I decided to give my room a bit of a tidy. It's hard to keep such a small space tidy when you have so much in it.

I wasn't expecting my doctor to come to see me today, but he appeared anyhow. He told me that the last sputum sample I had given had come back positive. However, it was only borderline positive. Although it was still technically a positive result, he seemed flexible about this. I'm not coughing, and the amount of TB bacilli in my sample is so small that the chances of me infecting anyone now must be minuscule.

The doctor has said that as soon as suitable accommodation has been found for me I can go. When he left I felt confused. Did I hear that right? Am I going to be free?

I sat in the corner of the room and cried. I felt near to breaking point. There had been no visits from the Psychologist for the last three weeks. My fear turned to frustration to elation and back again. I paced the room once more.

[Letter] Tuesday 10th October, 1995
Dear Sirs,

I was watching The James Whale Show *in the early hours about one 24-year-old man who may have to be kept in isolation for the rest of his life.*

I write to a prisoner on Death Row in Florida, USA – if it is possible, I would like to write to this poor man in isolation?

Yours Faithfully,

S.V, South Byfleet

[Diary] Tuesday 10ᵗʰ October, 1995

One of the doctors came to see me today with a letter from the Consultant. It read:

"I thought it wise to set out in writing our advice to you concerning possible discharge. The following instructions will apply for when you only have small amounts of acid-fast bacilli in your sputum.

You should sleep in a single room with the door closed at night and should spend the majority of your time inside. It is relatively safe for you to go out for short periods assuming you will not be in close contact with anyone for longer than a quarter of an hour or so. This means you will not be able, for example, to go to restaurants, clubs, or use public transport. The flat should be properly ventilated.

You will need to comply with daily direct observed therapy and will be advised to attend our out-patients' clinic once monthly. You should have no new social contacts and should not have contact with anyone who is HIV-positive or otherwise immuno-compromised. You should also not have any contact with pregnant women or children."

I was elated. It finally seemed like I was getting somewhere. They have told me I can go this Friday. All I need is one more test result. I don't care. It looks as though I'm definitely getting out of here, and that's enough for me.

The day passed, and at about 6.30pm one of the nurses came to see me. "I have got some news for you," he said. '*What now?*', I thought: I'd become so used to getting one piece of news immediately contradicted by another. He had been talking with the doctor who had received my latest test result from the lab.

My sputum smear test results had come back negative. I am no longer infectious!!

.

DIURNE - EPILOGUE

"Make it a rule of life never to regret and never to look back. Regret is an appalling waste of energy; you can't build on it; it's only for wallowing in."
The Letters of Katherine Mansfield

Instead of the celestial ball of light I was expecting to experience at the end of the tunnel after I'd exhaled my last breath, it was daylight that greeted me on Friday 13th October, 1995. The air was cool and I filled my tired lungs with it. Summer had been and gone. The leaves had turned brown and were falling on the pavement. The natural cycle of death and rebirth, soon the winter. The snow would come and then later melt. I knew deep down that spring and the green leaves would return. I had lost everything, my home, my partner and, to a degree, myself. I was unsure of who I was anymore and what would become of me. In that moment I knew that all any of us has is the space in between each breath we take.

I put the key into a front door I didn't recognize. It was only temporary accommodation, but it was mine for today.

A couple of months passed and I found somewhere to live permanently and gradually my new life came together. I took legal action against the hospital where I had contracted MDR-TB. We agreed an out-of-court settlement after about three years, only days before the case was due to be heard in the High Court of London. It had been scheduled for December 1st, 1998, World AIDS Day.

A new person was forged out of what happened in the room. It's taken time to get to know him. Paul Thorn today is quite different to Paul Mayho, the young, frightened man who found himself in a room 12ft by 10ft, being told that if he didn't die he would probably need to stay there for the rest of his life. Something happened in isolation that fundamentally changed me as a person, and I make no apologies for whom I've become. I have worked for many years in the HIV and TB arena and shall continue to do so until the job is done.

As I write this, it is 2018. Twenty-three years have passed since I contracted this lonely disease and it has been twenty years since I was cured of it. I spent three years on a grueling treatment regimen of toxic tablets and injections. Taking these drugs was worse than having the disease itself. The side effects of them had a catastrophic effect on me. Fortunately, I seem physically to have weathered them – many others are not so lucky.

This short book is not an attempt to romanticize TB in the historical 'consumptive literature' sense. Its purpose is to bring a more recent, personal account to readers that illustrates the crushing loneliness of having TB today.

Treating TB is more than a medical affair; it affects every facet of one's life. I tell my story to give new insight to the modern experience of having the disease and to highlight the plight of those around the world, right now, who are living with TB and without a voice. Many are, as you read these final pages, in isolation. It's not actually known how many there are. This, in itself, is a travesty; that the number of human beings in isolation isn't recorded – they are out of the way and no more than exist, sometimes forgotten for years. Tuberculosis is usually rendered non-infectious after a few weeks of treatment; MDR-TB may take a bit longer and can be treated in the community after the infectious stage. It's not necessary that so many have lost their liberty. There is another way.

There's no question in my mind that the Public Health strategy to address the global threat of TB has failed in most recent decades and continues to fail. Global statistics are disappointing at least, there is a lack of new diagnostic and treatment tools, and even the few new drugs we have are not being used widely because many in Public Health want to "protect the drug for the future".

This is the truth... TB and indeed MDR-TB are treatable and curable. However, many of the older drugs have severe side effects. We live in a world where some children and adults after TB and MDR-TB treatment are left deaf, blind, psychotic, and sometimes unable to leave their homes because they require constant oxygen, but this is considered a "treatment success" by the Public Health community because the sufferers have also been cured of TB and are therefore non-infectious to the abstract wider population. This doesn't have to be what "success" looks like. Any strategy to deal with the problem the world faces from *Mycobacterium tuberculosis* needs to have its roots in a human rights-based approach, a strategy that puts a person with TB and its drug-resistant variants at the centre of all activities associated in curing it to achieve the best possible outcome for everyone.

All people, wherever they are from in the world, should have access to the most sensitive diagnostic testing, the most effective medicines, and every effort should be made to maintain their dignity and freedom. No one must die because of TB in 2018, and yet it remains the biggest killer due to bacterial infection in the world.

This is Exhibit A, the primary evidence that the global Public Health strategy has been failing for years. We need more than words from politicians, their signature on a declaration. Those working in the TB arena need to stop being so fucking polite. Civil society needs to stop being so civil. We need to call out those in Public Health who are failing the most vulnerable and hold our governments to account. Promises are not enough. It is possible to 'end TB in our lifetimes', if there's the political will to do so.

"...for in the final analysis our most basic common link is that we all inhabit this small planet. We breathe the same air. We all cherish our children's futures, and we are all mortal."

John F. Kennedy, June 10th, 1963

This book has been published to mark the High-Level Meeting on Tuberculosis taking place at the United Nations in New York on Wednesday 26th September, 2018. World leaders and high-ranking officials will discuss TB and the global threat it presents. One only hopes that history will look back on this High-level Meeting as a 'game changer' in the fight against this ancient disease that still threatens our modern world today. This will only happen if the leaders of the nations of the world are truly united in their determination to "end TB in our lifetime". Their failure will mean millions more lives lost needlessly. If history shows this High-Level meeting not to be the turning point, then may it judge those who lead our nations accordingly.

Printed in Great Britain
by Amazon